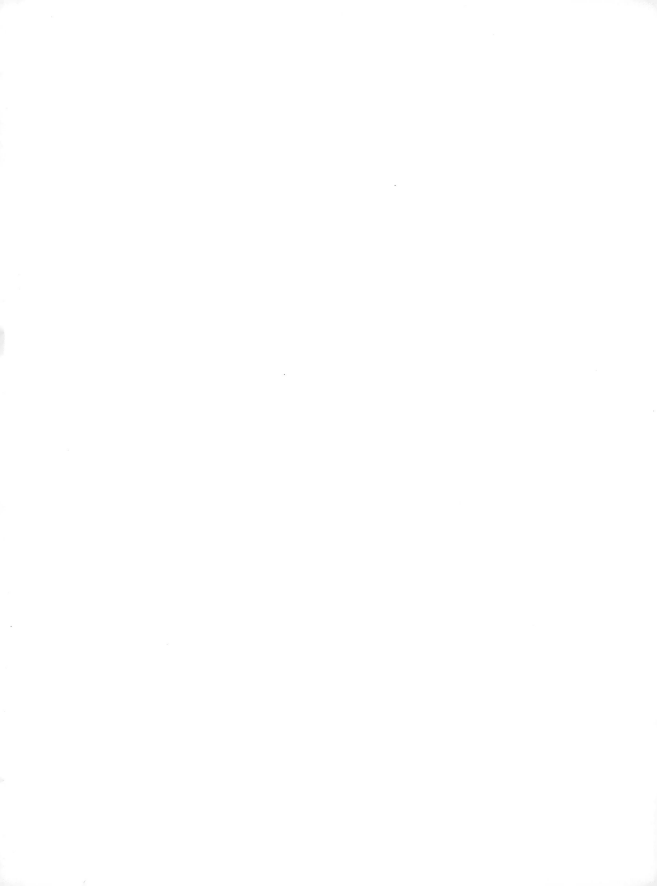

Understanding Masticatory Function in Unilateral Crossbites

For my father and mother,
who taught me about intellectual integrity,
which is the cornerstone of this book.

For Stefano and Federica, for putting up with such a "busy mom."

MGP

Understanding Masticatory Function in Unilateral Crossbites

Maria Grazia Piancino, MD, DDS, PhD

Researcher and Aggregate Professor – Orthognathodontics
Dental School International Research Center
Department of Surgical Sciences
University of Turin
Turin, Italy

Stephanos Kyrkanides, DDS, PhD

Dean
College of Dentistry
University of Kentucky
Lexington, KY, USA

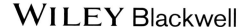

Contents

Foreword

This book's uniqueness lies in the fact that it studies malocclusion from a gnathological viewpoint, in terms of both diagnosis and treatment. The study of masticatory function includes gnathological principles that allow us to understand the functional aspects of malocclusion conditions and their effects on the entire stomatognathic system. A gnathological approach helps us understand the importance of selecting and applying treatments which respect overall physiological wellbeing.

Indeed, it is only through balanced and harmonious function that a developing system may grow healthily from a neurophysiological perspective, avoiding impairment and maintaining these results constantly throughout adulthood. Therefore, the final goal of early orthognathodontic treatment is to achieve (via the teeth) a rebalancing of function by following gnathological principles. The study of theories forwarded by respected scholars (from Gisi onwards) of the structure and function of the masticatory system and craniomaxillofacial area was extremely important for us.

During our studies we had the chance to understand the works of, as well as spend time with, B. McCollum, Ch. Stuart, H. Stallard, and P. K. Thomas (nicknamed "the immortals of Loma Linda University"), along with R. Lee, S. P. Ramfjord, T. Lundeen, and B. Jankelson. A special mention goes to R. Slavicek of the University of Vienna and A. Lewin of the University of Witwatersrand in Johannesburg, South Africa. The ideas and teachings of these scholars (on whose work our own is founded) were fundamental in the writing of this book about crossbite, thanks to their smart understanding of the risks and collateral effects as well as neuromuscular implications of the condition.

This is a matter studied and discussed by many but still deserving of further research, owing to the important and irreversible gnathological implications that we have learnt to identify thanks to the aforementioned experts. The knowledge gathered by research into mastication and then applied to the use of orthognathodontic devices before/after treatment has been essential in understanding the effect of occlusion on chewing cycles and the importance of respecting gnathological principles when selecting therapies.

The understanding and respect of these principles allowed the perfection over time of a therapy that for many years gave even better results than we could have predicted. Thanks to the study of masticatory function, many of these results became clearer, and they are described in this book in a precise and logical way (despite the complexity of the topic).

The project was not easy, and is the result of many years of research into the fields of orthognathodontics and masticatory function. I hope, above all, that this book can spark a change, a move towards a gnathological approach in the diagnosis and treatment of malocclusions, in light of the fact that the true goal of a medical dentistry field like orthognathodontics should be the functional balance and harmony of the stomatognathic system.

Pietro Bracco
University of Turin
Italy

Preface

Masticatory Function as a Reference Point

The study of malocclusion conditions and their relationship with masticatory function is of interest for the medical dentistry and the medical field in general. If one considers that malocclusions appear during the years of growth (i.e., during the psychophysical development of a child), the complexity and importance of the matter is clear. Owing to the difficulty even today of acquiring reliable studies and tools, the orthodontic field is more attracted and inundated with mechanical theories and related technological innovations that too often focus on dental shifting *tout court* without considering the functional outcomes.

Masticatory function is one of the oldest and most important phylogenetic functions for humans, both during childhood development and in adulthood, right through to old age. It requires precise coordination between dental occlusion, masticatory muscles, joint structures, and motor control. One of the malocclusions that undoubtedly affects mastication, with irreversible consequences once childhood development is complete, is that of crossbite.

This book focuses on the study of masticatory function, both in the event of physiological occlusion and in cases of pre and posttreatment of unilateral crossbite malocclusion, with descriptions and analysis of the clinical features of masticatory irregularity. This field is still considered rather as the "poor relation" of medicine and medical dentistry, in that it is rarely studied and often sidelined. However, in this day and age for most developed countries, a healthy and balanced masticatory function is fundamental in contributing to a good social life and relations and combating stress.

The best-known "players" in mastication are the teeth. Teeth are phylogenetic ancient structures and may no longer be a vital organ of survival for humans, as they are for animals. They still show very precise neural connections and are essential in terms of optimal physiological functioning. In other words, balanced dental occlusion and healthy masticatory function play an important part in enhancing our quality of life. Certainly, the study of mastication as described here is closely linked to orthognathodontic diagnoses and treatment.

Three experts have guided me in said study, without whom this research would never have taken place. I owe them my eternal esteem and admiration:

Arthur Lewin (University of the Witwatersrand, South Africa), a true friend, who ignited the first spark of an idea for this research project with his teaching on the clinical significance of chewing pattern and his open-minded approach that went beyond the traditional mathematical–statistic constraints of masticatory study.

Giuseppe Anastasi (University of Messina, Italy), with whom I shared some of the most exciting moments of the research project. Thanks to his intelligence, open mind, and determination, the molecular and functional magnetic resonance imaging (fMRI) proof of gnathographic and electromyographic clinical results of mastication were collected. He passed on to me his enthusiasm for the study of neural control, without which it would be impossible to understand masticatory function.

And last but not least, Pietro Bracco (University of Turin, Italy), my mentor forever, from whom I learnt the gnathological rules of coherent and physiological orthognathodontics. His clinical imprint has been fundamental both in the research process and in my professional and teaching life.

I owe these three men my sincere gratitude for having taught me to reason in physiological and gnathological terms (i.e. in terms of masticatory function), an approach, which lies at the base of this book.

A Consistent Reasoning from Diagnosis to Therapy

The book is divided into two main parts. The first is dedicated to mastication, its understanding and clinical importance of research results achieved with electrognathography and electromyography over years, and confirmed unequivocally by histological and morphology (as well as fMRI) studies of the masticatory muscles. The second, based on the results of the first, is dedicated to actions and effects and, above all, to functional and gnathological reasons for the use of the Function Generating Bite appliance, which corrects not only teeth, but especially masticatory function, avoiding basal and dental traumatisms and respecting biology and physiology of the structures.

The aim of this book is to give the reader (students or doctors or enthusiasts) a physiological and biological overview of the stomatognathic system, evidence-based on reliable scientific results and, for the first time, a consistent reasoning from diagnosis through therapy. This means that, to respect the biology and physiology of the stomatognathic system, structural and denta traumatic therapies are not coherent while the proposed treatment is established on the basis of functional and gnathological principles. To acquire a new approach to the subject, it is necessary (as always) to maintain an open mind and make a small effort to understanding and memorizing the various features – this effort will be amply repaid by the acquired learning of a logical sequence from diagnosis to therapy, also with useful practical aspects.

To sum up, knowing that the stomatognathic system is a vital factor in the quality of life for each and every one of us, it is our hope that this book will introduce a truly new approach to "curing" (in medical terms) one of the most important district of the human body for a balanced living.

Maria Grazia Piancino

How to Use This Book

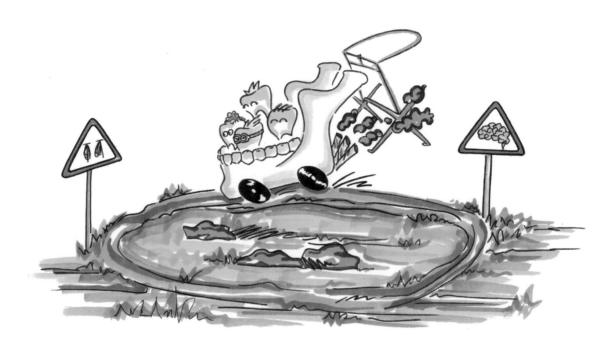

This book brings together the lecture notes of courses imparted to students at the postgraduate School of Orthognathodontics and at the degree course in Dentistry and Prosthodontics at the University of Turin, Italy. It is the result of more than 20 years of study and research, with the contributions of students, patients, professionals, bio-engineers, and dedicated scholars. The original source material (i.e., the lessons themselves) has influenced the writing of this book, and it is the pictures and diagrams that lead the reader through a voyage of discovery exploiting the visual memory where the final objective is understanding the importance of therapeutical respect for the stomatognathic system's physiology, biology, and memory function. We believe that the use of visual memory and progressive "familiarity" with the subject (as opposed to vice versa) helps make this book a simple aid to study, and a source of immediate and stimulating comprehension and reference of the complex subject of masticatory function. Its links to growth and orthognathodontics represent one of the most fascinating areas of medicine and dentistry.

Acknowledgments

Many people have contributed, both directly and indirectly, to this book and research.

I would like to give a special mention to Dr Teresa Vallelonga (University of Turin, Italy), not only for the enormous amount of work she contributed to the production of this book, but also for the professional support and effort constantly demonstrated during the long years of research that ran parallel to the book's creation. I greatly appreciated her determination even during very busy times; this book will remain permanently linked to the two mascots, Maria Chiara and Giacomo.

I am equally grateful to my co-author, Stephanos Kyrkanides (University of Kentucky, USA), who is my "overseas" support – his European roots combined with his US professional training and incredible mental openness were fundamental for the explanation of such a complex topic as mastication in orthognathodontic terms, and for the realization of this book. I owe him my sincere gratitude.

Special thanks go to Prof Ezio Ghigo (Univeristy of Turin, Italy) for his support and mentorship in transmitting to me an enthusiasm for the idea of this book, which proved so necessary to me during its writing. A huge thank-you, with respect and affection.

My gratitude also goes to bioengineers Prof Dario Farina and Prof Deborah Falla (University of Goettingen, Germany) and Dr Andrea Merlo (Polytechnic of Turin, Italy) for the creation of the data analysis software without which a reliable research project into mastication would never have been possible.

Many thanks to Prof Guglielmo Ramieri and Dr Francesca Bianchi (University of Turin, Italy) for the special collaboration in the maxillo-facial research studies.

Thank you also to Prof Placido Bramanti (University of Messina, Italy) for his availability with the magnetic resonance imaging and to Prof Giuseppina Cutroneo (University of Messina, Italy) for the valuable morphological evaluation.

I wish to thank Dr Luca Cortina for his availability and great talent that I very much appreciated in the preparation of images and charts, Dr Corrado De Biase for managing the bibliography section, Dr Maria Grazia Incardona for her help in the management of the images of cases, Dr Luigi Sordella for the management of the images, and the valuable staff in the offices of Dr Mario Serra and Dr Luca Bava for their collaboration and for putting up with such a busy orthognathodontist.

My sincere gratitude goes to the staff at Wiley who helped bring this book to completion and who supported me throughout this entire project: Rick Blanchette, Nick Morgan, Catriona Cooper, Teri Jensen, and Jennifer Seward; and to the project manager Aileen Castell and the copy editor Peter Lewis.

A special thank you to Victoria Clifford for quick and professional translation services.

Last but not least, thanks to all our undergraduate and postgraduate students of the University of Turin and to the professionals for their enthusiasm and for providing fundamental contributions over time to the acquisition, processing, and recording of data, particularly to Dr Francesca Talpone for her care and the safekeeping of the research materials, especially in the initial, threatened stages of this project.

Maria Grazia Piancino

Chapter 1

Introductory Explanation of Masticatory Function

Contents

Understanding Masticatory Function in Unilateral Crossbites, First Edition. Maria Grazia Piancino and Stephanos Kyrkanides.
© 2016 John Wiley & Sons, Inc. Published 2016 by John Wiley & Sons, Inc.

1.1 Introduction

Mastication is one of the most important functions of the stomatognathic system. *It is a highly coordinated neuromuscular operation and features rapid mandibular movements* that demand continual modulation and adaptation to load. The nervous system, peripheral receptors (which determine sensory input), and the masticatory muscles (which produce the response from the brain and adaptation of movement) are continually involved during mastication. This is a complex process and *plays a fundamental role in the quality of life for patients during childhood, maturity, and old age.*

Mastication is *a rhythmic and phylogenetically ancient movement*. The best-known players in this process are the teeth; these are no longer a vital organ for humans (as they are for animals, for example), but they are still of fundamental importance both in terms of healthy functioning of the stomatognathic system and for social relationships. In fact, the peripheral input arriving from the periodontal receptors of teeth is numerically concentrated, sensitive, highly specialized, and extremely fast in reaching the neural centers allocated to masticatory control. Experimental studies on the topic have identified the mechanisms in animals during phylogenetic development that maintain and control the chewing cycles, mechanisms that are extremely precise in humans too. However, it is the cerebral cortex – which is so developed in human beings that it takes up half of the brain area – that controls the chewing pattern.

At this point, the "clinical physiopathology of masticatory function" becomes of specific interest, particularly the search to link masticatory function with dental occlusion, structural and neuromuscular structures, and the whole brain (Figure 1.1). This scientific interest emerged and was developed during the 1980s at the School of Orthognathic Studies in the University of Turin under

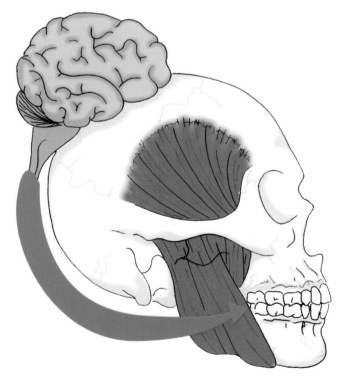

Figure 1.1 Linking masticatory function with dental occlusion, cranial structure, and neuromuscular activity.

the leadership of Professor P. Bracco. From the very outset, he focused on a functional, multidisciplinary, and especially gnathological approach to the diagnosis and therapy of malocclusions. The study and comprehension of masticatory function was supported by this underlying methodology, without which the research carried out would have been limited to the simple publication of statistical results without any true contribution being made to the improvement of diagnostic and therapeutic procedures. Such contribution is, however, the true objective of all research.

In the fields of orthognathics and prosthetics, the study of occlusion is extremely important, particularly as the correlation between "occlusion" (involving the teeth of upper and lower dental arches), function, aesthetics, and social relationships becomes increasingly acknowledged. An understanding of the relationships between dental occlusion and neural control has been improved beyond question by gnathological knowledge of occlusion (Figure 1.2). It was also clear from very early on that, in order to understand and establish a meaningful clinical study, the gnathological base would have to be supported by an understanding of neurology. The concepts of functional occlusion and neuromuscular control are very close to the question of medical treatment of the psychophysical aspect of humans. This concept is clearly expressed in Springer's *International Journal of Stomatology and Occlusion Medicine*, a title created by

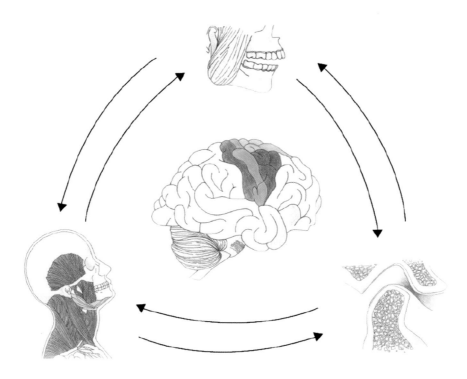

Figure 1.2 The stomatognathic system: relationships between dental occlusion, temporomandibular joint (TMJ) and neuromuscular control. *Source for the muscles:* redrawn from Neff (1999). *Source for the brain:* Purves *et al.* (2000). Reproduced with the permission of Sinauer Associates.

Professor R. Slavicek, one of the most important and dedicated modern-day gnathologists. Dentistry deals with one of the most refined anatomical areas of the body from a neuromuscular point of view – it has an incredible ability to adapt, which, instead of being abused, should be studied and understood in all its physiological aspects in order to allow treatments, "cures" even, that improve its functioning and, consequently, the general psychophysical health of the patient. We hope, then, that the study of mastication can help achieve this objective.

The information gathered from chewing patterns is important in diagnosing the functional condition of the patient; for example, the repetition and variability of mandibular movement, neuromuscular coordination between the two sides, or the ability to adapt to load while chewing a hard bolus. As the brain is entirely engaged during chewing, the importance of this study from a clinical point of view is clear, but the technical, statistical–mathematical, and numeric difficulties have meant that only professionals working specifically in this field have been involved in the research so far. One aspect of evolution is to simplify complex processes, and this is the aim of this book, a first step in this direction. The fine-tuning of functional magnetic resonance imaging (fMRI) has allowed the study of neural control in humans, which we hope will permit us to better understand the functioning of the central nervous system.

The study of masticatory function began at the University of Turin in the 1980s, when the first devices for recording human chewing patterns were produced and sold. The necessary hardware and software were developed and fine-tuned over many years, thanks to the fundamental and collaborative work of the bioengineers Professor D. Farina and Dr A. Merlo. We will later look at the intrinsic difficulties encountered in the study of functional movement from a statistical–mathematical point of view, which were overcome thanks to the skill and effort of these professionals – without their contribution, none of the results later achieved would have been possible. Not only the bioengineers, but also many researchers, professionals, students, and volunteers dedicated their time and energy to this research, even during the period when its clinical significance was still unclear. We believe it important to underline this contribution to clinical research, which requires a true and homogeneous team who all offer hard work and intellectual integrity, albeit in different capacities. These elements, along with a smidgeon of good luck (or, rather, the open-minded approach necessary to identify an important finding amongst millions of others) are essential in achieving scientifically valid and sound results. True research (which presupposes the objective of increasing and developing knowledge) requires skill and passion, as opposed to personal interests connected to obscure indexes of scientific impact. Using research results that have clarified the correlation between masticatory function and occlusion as a starting point, two new directions have emerged thanks to a collaborative partnership between Professor G. Anastasi (University of Messina Italy) and Professor P. Bramanti (IRCCS Centro Neurolesi "Bonino Pulejo," Messina, Italy) – the study in fMRI of neural control during chewing and the histological and biomolecular study of the sarcoglycan–integrin system of the masseter muscle:

1. *The use of fMRI has allowed the study of neural control in human chewing* (Figure 1.3) and represents a step forward in the correlated research not only in dentistry but also, and principally, at a neurological level because it has permitted us to widen our knowledge about the central nervous system via the study of a complex automatism i.e., mastication. Both neural control of mastication and the phenomenon of occlusion differ greatly in their characteristics with regard to human beings as opposed to most species of animals (particularly small laboratory animals). Thus, the study of mastication is now moving beyond the confines of dentistry, the area in which it started, to develop within the field of human neurology and contribute, hopefully, to the understanding of much more serious and debilitating conditions than malocclusion.

2. *The morphological and biomolecular aspects of masticatory muscles are currently a focus of interest*. Despite the fact that considerable information exists, various questions still remain

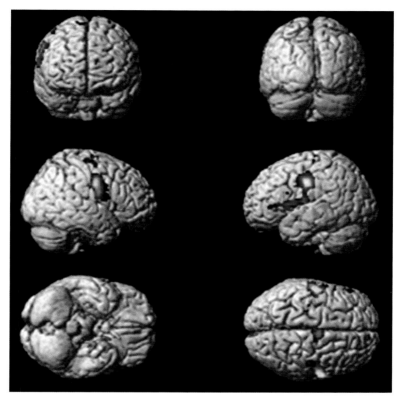

Figure 1.3 Functional magnetic resonance has allowed the study of neural control during masticatory function. *Source:* Bracco *et al.* (2010). Reproduced with the permission of Maney Publishing.

about these muscles that are characterized by special features, both macroscopic and microscopic. However, if the characteristics of a complex muscle like the masseter are to be understood well, it is necessary that there be a strict correlation with the clinical features of masticatory function.

We have outlined these innovative aspects of the study of masticatory function in order to introduce the reader to the topic with an open mind, putting aside preconceptions and convictions that in no way aid true and in-depth understanding of the overall subject.

We wish to underline above all the fact that the stomatognathic system's capacity for "functional compensation" cannot be used as an excuse to justify all and any type of therapy. It is true that *the stomatognathic system possesses remarkable (although restricted) compensatory capacities, but it is also the case that, in general, it has no autocorrection capacity.* This means that, during life, the compensations made will add up and overlap, also with those of poorly selected therapies, to the point where the system is unbalanced and then recovery becomes extremely difficult due to the need for multifactor and multidisciplinary solutions.

The only way to avoid such an imbalance is to prevent it – this is why we must try, *using the appropriate treatment, to restore ideal physiological conditions in each patient* (Figure 1.4). A working knowledge of ideal functioning conditions for each human is important if the right therapeutic cure is to be selected, without adverse side effects that may at times remain hidden, undiagnosed,

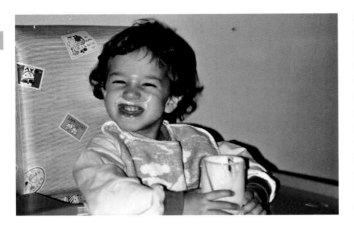

Figure 1.4   The beginning of masticatory function.

or impossible to diagnose. The additional peripheral information (on which subliminal information is based) activates an unconscious muscle reaction, at times well balanced but at other times causing unexplained tiredness and/or acute or chronic craniofacial pain. If we also add stress to this list (part of our emotional make-up that often unburdens itself unconsciously onto the stomatognathic system), it is easy to understand how, over time (and as the compensatory actions amass), the system can reach a point of no return. *The chances of correction (as opposed to compensation) during the initial phase are considerable if a correct diagnosis and a correct physiological therapy are made.* But once a phase of compensation is initiated, due to the malocclusion per se or to a traumatic and non physiological therapy the situation is much more difficult, as it becomes multifactor and multidisciplinary, and no feasible solution may remain. Thus, we have to make every effort possible to avoid this phase of imbalance by intervening promptly to correct the occlusal and functional disease with treatments appropriate to physiological and biological conditions. In fact, compensation is evoked to preserve fully functioning order in the best way possible, but at times this may produce collateral damage in the long term. Many discussions, opinions, and arguments have been forwarded on this question, but it is the physiological aspect, not the philosophy of the issue, that interests us. And *the physiology can only be studied, understood, known, and respected*.

The topic is extremely complex and, unfortunately, we do not yet have the right diagnostic means available to fully understand the limits of the stomatognathic system's compensatory function. Therein lies the real aim of this book: *to provide the reader with simple means for a general comprehension (supported by reliable scientific results) of mastication, in order to enable him/her to choose respectful therapies and treatments*. We hope that the book will help professionals in various sectors (including orthodontists, dentists, neurologists, psychiatrists, pediatricians, rehabilitation physicians, physiotherapists, osteopaths, and sports coaches) to understand the causes, development, and consequences of malocclusion in childhood and maturity, in order to adopt and refine therapies that take both physiology and biology into consideration. To achieve this aim from a practical and not simply theoretic point of view, and *to learn how to "think physiologically,"* we need to put aside all our preconceptions and old ways of thinking to make a slight initial effort to study this new subject. Orthognathodontics, just like any other profession, is in continual evolution, and *it is currently of clinical relevance in successful orthodontic or prosthetic treatments to consider not only the repositioning or substitution of teeth within the dental arches, but also, and above all, the effects of treatment on the functional working of the masticatory system*.

1.2 The study of masticatory function

It is now time *to describe briefly the intrinsic difficulties in the study of mastication*, from both technological and clinical points of view, in order to show the reader the evolution, benefits, and limits of the research. Mastication is a complex rhythmic movement that has been refined over millions of years in the animal world and is characterized by precise and reliable neuromuscular control. Thus, the study of this function is extremely complex and requires not only *advanced technological tools, but also clinical experience and skill*. Furthermore, intellectual integrity is vital, which is why we have published these results only after confirmation at least twice by different groups of researchers treating different patients. Clinical experience, then, is the basis of research planning in order to have a logical plan of action with its roots in physiology – when the research plan is not underpinned by knowledge and experience, there is a danger of producing untrustworthy results. One of the most common defects in the literature is in regard to the nonhomogeneous nature or inaccurate selection of samples where homogeneity is a vital factor. Technological evolution and compliance have also played an important ongoing role.

As a result of the discrepancy between technological resources and clinical comprehension, there was an initial period of confusion that was only resolved with many years of research and effort to gain reliable data. In the 1980s, computers were certainly not so advanced as nowadays, but they could still supply long lists of numbers tracking the movement of the mandible in the three planes. In this initial painstaking phase, all effort was focused on discovering how and in what length of time data could be collected, on the alignment and successive processing of data from different sources, and on the instructions to technicians involved in data collection so that they could record cases reliably. In other words, this period concentrated on resolving solely technical issues, in order to tackle the true question of which and how many of these machine-generated numbers could be used in clinical research. Perfecting the pathognomonic framework was a lengthy and arduous process, closely linked to the technological evolution of hardware and software. In particular, the relevant software was totally rewritten and adapted to the current clinical and technological progress. This took place following an in-depth study alongside bioengineers because it was clear from the start that the study of masticatory function was badly served by the laws of mathematics and statistics. In fact, as chewing patterns are characterized (in physiological conditions) by a balance of repetition and variability, it is difficult to link this study to the mathematical–statistic laws that the international scientific community holds dear. For this reason, much attention was paid to refining a software program that is suitable for the processing of collected data.

The software currently being used in research allows a reliable reading of basic data of chewing patterns and muscular activity, which will be described in Chapters 2 and 3. However, it is necessary to point out that masticatory function cannot be compared with a hemochemical test – to be correctly analyzed, *it needs to be linked to clinical, occlusal, cranial, articular, muscular, and, in some cases, emotive characteristics* of the patient, as previously mentioned. The dentistry profession is obviously interested in the relationships between occlusion (or malocclusion) and chewing patterns. However, as humans are psychophysical beings, the emotive aspect can in some cases become a significant factor, influencing not only the pattern but also the entire motor control of the jaw movement. Thus, it is clear that a multidisciplinary approach to this study is essential, with expertise from various fields being integrated for maximum efficiency.

We will now dedicate a few lines to some key authors in the field who have influenced the work described in this book. Possibly for the reasons outlined above, the research and study of mastication have been awarded little attention, generally by just a handful of international authors. First, we will give a brief description of the significance of early research studies into the topic, looking more closely at those which influenced current understanding of chewing patterns.

J. Ahlgren, 1960–1970: one of the first scholars of chewing patterns in humans. He studied mandibular jaw movement in its entirety, identifying some typical patterns (Ahlgren, 1967).

E. Moller 1960–1970: he carried out an electromyographic (EMG) study of the masseter and temporal muscles of mastication during chewing in order to identify the characteristics of masticatory muscle coordination, a vital factor in understanding neuromuscular control of chewing kinetics (Moller, 1966).

These two authors carried out their studies without the possibility of analyzing mandibular kinetic movement and EMG activity simultaneously. However, despite the limited technology of their age, their results demonstrate high levels of awareness of the issues involved and clinical experience.

Y. Kawamura 1970–1980: the author of *Physiology of Mastication*, a book that joined a few other texts in describing neuromuscular control of chewing patterns based on experimental research of the time (Kawamura, 1974).

C. H. Gibbs and A. Lundeen 1980–1990: these scholars studied chewing patterns using the "case gnathic replicator," an unwieldy device that was difficult to use and required considerable effort but which allowed the collection of data that are still considered accurate and valid today. Moreover, the device succeeded in registering masticatory movement at interincisive, bilateral molar, and bilateral articular levels. These authors described chewing cycles with mathematic precision, making an important contribution to the understanding of masticatory function. Their vital research results are described in Chapter 2 (Lundeen and Gibbs, 1982).

A. Lewin 1985: Lewin focused on the study of mastication in the same period as Gibbs (1989–1990), laying the foundations for diagnostic analysis today. He studied chewing patterns with the "Sirognathograph," a less invasive tool than the case gnathic replicator that also proved easier to use. Thanks to his experience and intuition, Lewin was able to identify the clinical features of chewing patterns, which were then confirmed by further studies and are outlined in Chapter 2 (Lewin, 1985). He is a cornerstone in the field.

J. P. Lund 1970–1990: carried out basic research on the topic and was the first to prove the existence of the central pattern generator (masticatory-like rhythmic bursting in NVsnpr neurons) in the brainstem. This was a vital step in understanding neural control of mastication (Dellow and Lund, 1971; Bernier *et al.*, 2010).

A. Woda 1984: on the basis of research carried out on mastication, he performed an in-depth study into the characteristics of receptors and reflexes of the stomatognathic system, and then outlined their clinical significance (Woda, 1984; Witter *et al.*, 2013). V. F. Ferrario focused on the study of the masticatory muscles coordination during chewing (Ferrario and Sforza, 1996). B. J. Sessle, 1980–1990, studied mastication from an experimental point of view, particularly in non-human primate species (Nakamura and Sessle, 1990). Y. Nakamura 1980–1990: published a book on mastication, gathering together experimental studies referred to in a Tokyo congress in 1990 (Nakamura and Sessle, 1990). K. Takada 1996: developed a system to calculate the masseter muscle's "silent period" during mastication (Takada *et al.*, 1992).

The key research authors that this book makes reference to are C. H. Gibbs and A. Lewin, who conducted their research studies with very different tools from both conceptual and practical points of view (case gnathic replicator and Sirognathograph). They were also very distant geographically, coming from the USA and South Africa, but were active during the same time period (1980–1990). Current research on chewing cycles still today refers to these authors' results and concepts, reconfirming their validity.

1.2.1 The case gnathic replicator

The American researcher Gibbs (1985, USA) developed the first machine designed not only to record human mandibular movement but also to reproduce said movement later. The process involved a heavy, unwieldy, and invasive device, but it had a huge advantage over previous methods in that it allowed the recording and (even more importantly) the reproduction of chewing patterns in plaster models of the dental arches, controlled by six small servomotors for precise and reliable results (Figure 1.5).

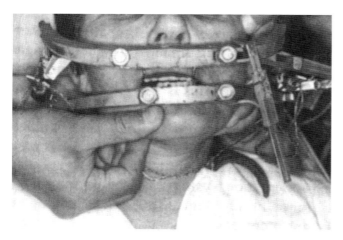

Figure 1.5   Multiple sensor array of Case Gnathic Replicator. *Source:* Lundeen and Gibbs (1982). Reproduced with permission from Elsevier.

Following their research study, Gibbs and Lundeen were able to produce literature on *chewing cycles at the interincisive level and at the molars on the right and left, as well as on bilateral temporomandibular movement*. Their work clarified the process of condylar movement during mastication. At that time, the use of axiographic tracing of TMJ movement was common (opening, closing, protrusion right and left-hand mediotrusion). Great astonishment greeted the discovery that, during mastication, the opening and closing patterns of the condyle on the bolus-loaded side are different to those of the contralateral. This, in fact, meant that at no point in mastication or in any masticatory movement was the position of the condylar axis the point of reference, as it was for all gnathology and dentistry study.

Given the complexity of the device involved, Gibbs's study was carried out on a limited number of patients and, despite the author's intentions, he never managed to make the device feasible for larger-scale studies. However, as already stated, the results obtained are important and still considered valid today (Lundeen and Gibbs, 1982).

1.2.2 The Sirognathograph

At the same time that Gibbs was developing the case gnathic replicator, Lewin (1985, South Africa) was perfecting his Sirognathograph, produced by Siemens (Germany). This was a much simpler piece of equipment to use, but, as a result, was able to produce less data than Gibbs's case gnathic replicator. Lewin's device records *the movement from one point of the mandible*, using a small magnet attached labially between the lower central incisors. The advantage of this method lies in the fact that it is less invasive, both regarding the stomatognathic system in general and the occlusion itself. The weight of the Sirognathograph antenna frame on the head and neck was an initial problem (Figure 1.6) but this problem was later resolved with increasingly advanced technology. It is also easier to use, allowing more cases to be studied (an important factor in developing clinical analysis of chewing patterns). The contribution that Lewin made to clinical analysis and clarity of

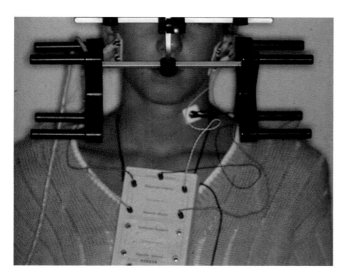

Figure 1.6   Multiple sensor array of the Sirognathograph (Siemens, Germany).

ideas on the protocol for recording chewing function remains fundamental in the research field even today, as his ideas and intuition are continually reconfirmed with more refined tools (Lewin, 1985). The research reported in this book is based on his teaching and guidelines.

1.3 The evolution of electrognathography and electromyography

While case histories, objective clinical examinations, experience, and diagnostic skill of doctors and dentists are essential elements in both professions, the use of advanced technological equipment permits the collection of clinical data that would not otherwise be possible. In particular, for mastication, although it is initially difficult to acquire this data and even more difficult to analyze it, great effort has been put into the development of hardware and software even when many researchers still openly criticized the use of diagnostic tools, claiming that clinical tests were more than sufficient for a correct diagnosis. We now know this is not true – whilst in no way diminishing the importance of clinical tests, the very fact of knowing the characteristics and correct or incorrect functioning of mastication, as well as being able to check post-treatment alteration, is important in the choice of corrective treatment from anatomic and mechanistic points of view and for the restoration of masticatory function in both evolutionary and growth phases. Here, we will outline *the evolution of electrognathography* to explain how the recording of such a process, *whilst seeming relatively simple, in fact required a lengthy and careful process to develop a valid and reliable tool that is also practical and easy to use*. This objective was reached along with the clinical analysis of results that, for some types of malocclusion, is today finally clear and scientifically demonstrated.

1.3.1 Plotted masticatory cycles

This book is based on research results that were initially gathered with the use of the Sirognathograph, developed by A. Lewin and produced and sold in the 1980s by the German company Siemens (Figures 1.7 and 1.8). This device recorded the movements of a magnet which was inserted labially in the lower midpoint of central incisors, and used an antenna frame with multiple sensors to track the motion of the magnet. At first, the Sirognathograph was not connected to a computer or EMG equipment. Connected to a plotter, it reproduced the mandibular movement of single chewing cycles in the three planes (frontal, sagittal, and transverse), but it

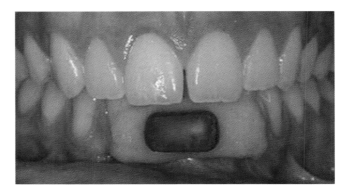

Figure 1.7   Magnet of the Sirognathograph.

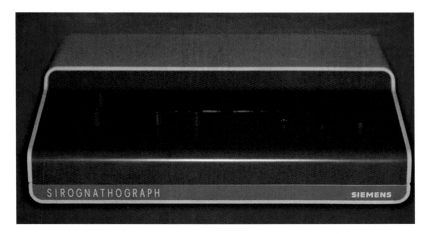

Figure 1.8   Sirognathograph.

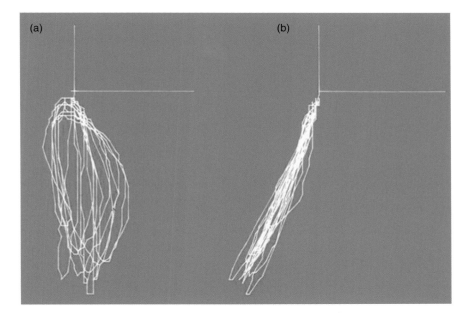

Figure 1.9   Single chewing cycles superimposed, in the frontal (a) and sagittal (b) planes recorded with Sirognathograph and reproduced with a plotter.

was impossible to process or archive any of the collected data (Figures 1.9 and 1.10). Plotting took around 30 min and demanded the constant presence of a technician to change the sheets. Furthermore, it was not possible to gain any information on masticatory muscle activity as the gathering of kinematic and EMG data was still problematic from a technological point of view; thus, in that period, the two processes (study of muscle activity and kinematic recording of mandibular movement) were carried out independently of one another. *The need for computerized*

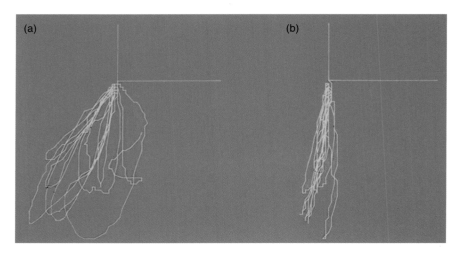

(a) (b)

Figure 1.10   Single chewing cycles superimposed in the frontal (a) and sagittal (b) planes.

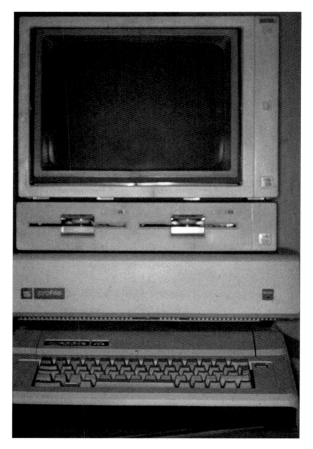

Figure 1.11   The computer connected to the Sirognathograph.

analysis of the complex masticatory function was soon obvious, and thanks to technological progress the Sirognathograph was soon linked up to an IBM computer.

1.3.2 1983: Early computer processing of plotted data on chewing cycles

The use of electrognathographic equipment for medical purposes allows the collection of large amounts of numeric data, but it also poses the problem of the difficulty of clinical analysis of said data. However, the need to process and record the numeric data on chewing cycles led to the connection of the Sirognathograph to a computer in 1986 (Figures 1.11, 1.12). The aim was to obtain the average chewing pattern, with the printing of charts and recorded data storage (Bracco *et al.*, 1990). The development of statistical and mathematical formulae to identify the average cycle (typical of the real chewing pattern in patients) required great effort and close collaboration with a valuable bioengineer E. Fabris. The difficulty of statistical–mathematical analysis of chewing cycles lies in the variability of the patterns, which is an intrinsic and fundamental feature in physiological conditions. However,

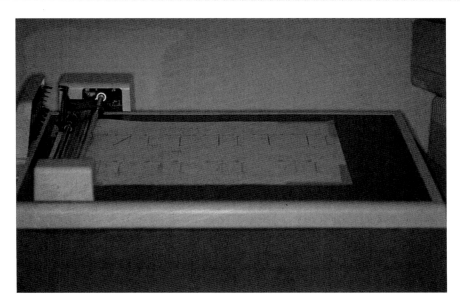

Figure 1.12   The plotter connected to the Sirognathograph

another equally important characteristic is the repetition of patterns, which is easily identi-fied by customized software. It was necessary to rewrite the program a number of times to apply the correct statistical–mathematical laws most appropriate to the intrinsic variability and repetition of masticatory patterns.

The first version of the program produced a graph of the average cycle on the frontal, sagittal, and transversal planes and the average duration time, allowing computerized data storage or printouts of data with significant savings of time and money. Also, thanks to computerization, it was possible to introduce the use of colors to distinguish patterns by using blue to represent opening and red for closing – this was a huge step forward in the understanding of masticatory patterns from a diagnostic point of view. The computer program was extremely advanced in comparison with our ability to interpret the results.

1.3.3 1986: First recording of chewing cycles in alignment with electromyography of the masseter and anterior temporalis muscles – customization of software

One important innovation for the reading and understanding of chewing cycles was surely the recording of EMG activity of the four masticatory muscles aligned to mandibular kinetic motion (Figures 1.8 and 1.15).

Only four of the eight masticatory muscles can be recorded with surface electrodes (right and left masseters, and right and left anterior temporalis). The other four (medial and lateral pterygoids) are detectable only by needle EMG recording, which is not suitable for the pur-poses of studying mastication. However, the different role of the masseters compared with the anterior temporalis muscles allows us to collect significant data that can help us understand the neuromuscular control of masticatory function. To this end, *it is necessary to clarify that the clinical importance of muscular activity during mastication is not so much connected to absolute EMG values, which are extremely sensitive to individual variables, as to the evaluation of muscle*

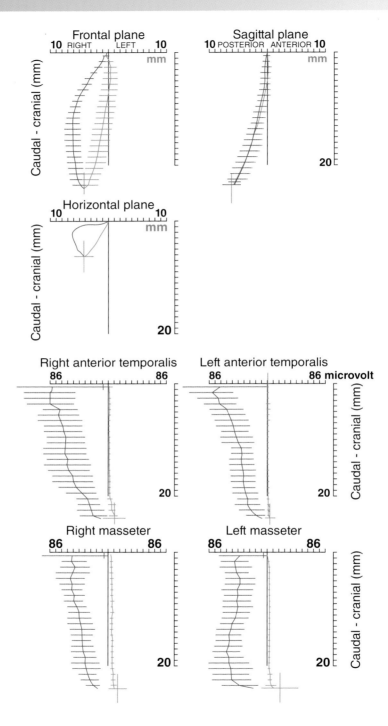

Figure 1.13 First plots of mandibular kinetic movement in frontal, sagittal, and horizontal planes (top) aligned with electromyography envelope plotted versus the vertical jaw displacement, of right and left anterior temporalis muscles and right and left masseters (bottom). Red tracings: opening; blue tracings: closing.

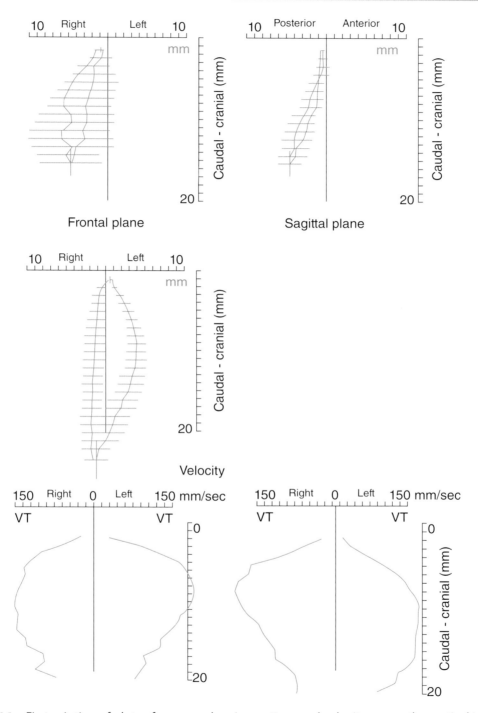

Figure 1.14 First printing of plots of average chewing pattern and velocity versus the vertical jaw displacement. Red tracings: opening; blue tracing: closing.

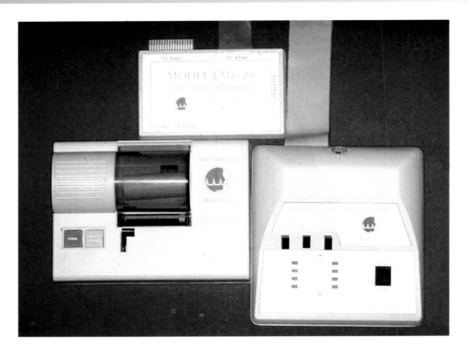

Figure 1.15 Electromyograph preamplifier (Myotronics, Tukwila, WA, USA).

coordination on the two sides. It is true that the reliability of EMG evaluation of these muscles has been confirmed (if carried out correctly), but it is necessary to look at coordination between the muscles during the study of masticatory function.

From a technical point of view, this evolution called for extremely advanced technological and resources considering the time in which it took place (Bracco *et al.*, 1999). The EMG recording of muscular activity aligned with mandibular kinetic movement represented an important step forward in clinical comprehension and diagnostic analysis of mastication in both physiological and pathological conditions (Figures 1.13, 1.14, and 1.15).

In order to be completely reliable, the study of muscular activity during mastication requires a huge amount of data. Individual variables in EMG activity is an intrinsic feature of mastication, whilst muscle coordination is an objective point of reference. The statistical evaluation of patients with *accurately identified malocclusions* (from a functional viewpoint) allows the identification of *pathognomonic EMG features*. Understanding neuromuscular activity and coordination between the muscles on the side of the bolus and contralateral muscle during mastication of hard and soft boluses is of fundamental clinical importance for the correct treatment of both youngsters and adults.

1.3.4 1992: Replacement of the Sirognathograph with a customized K6-I kinesiograph instrument – rewriting of the software

A further technological innovation took place when the Sirognathograph was replaced with the K6-I Myotronics kinesiograph (Tukwila, WA, USA). This move was imposed by circumstance rather than by choice (as opposed to the actively sought selection of EMG), due to the decision of Siemens in the 1990s to stop producing the Sirognathograph. Owing to its similar features, the K6-I Myotronics kinesiograph was chosen as a substitute (Figures 1.16 and 1.17).

The K6-I system was based on the same principles for recording mandibular movement and also offered the possibility of recording muscle activity of the four, aligned, masticatory muscles. The improvement resided in the more precise recording of movement and, above all, in the reduced invasiveness of the device thanks to its lighter weight and more anatomically friendly shape of the recording structure. However, from a software point of view, it was now practically back to square one!

The K6-I required the insertion of powerful hardware boards into a PC. The system unit had to be laid horizontally to prevent the large K6 boards touching other parts of the computer and damaging them. Both the antenna and the preamplifier were connected to the desktop PC and the equipment could not be moved in any way. The K6-I software was not originally developed for chewing cycle analysis, and so it was necessary to adapt the system with personalized software as well as writing

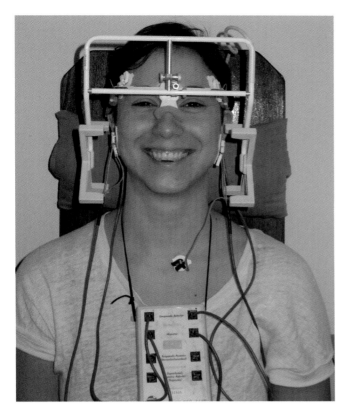

Figure 1.16 Multiple-sensor lightweight array of the kinesiograph (Myotronics, Tukwila, WA, USA).

new software for processing. It was the period of IT experts and it resulted in a transition software (Figures 1.16 and 1.18).

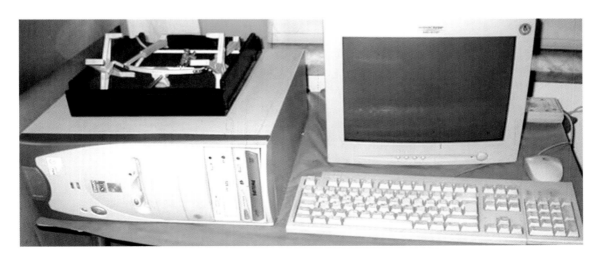

Figure 1.17 K6-I kinesiograph (Myotronics, Tukwila, WA, USA).

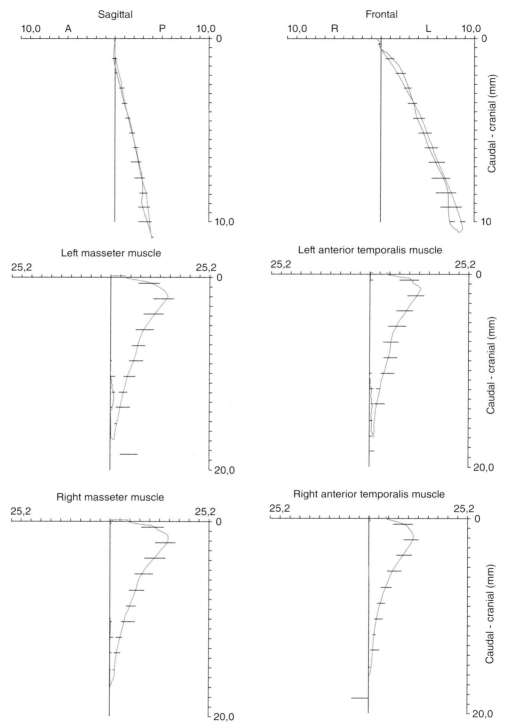

Figure 1.18 Prints of mandibular kinetic movement in frontal and sagittal planes (*top*) aligned with electromyography recordings of right and left anterior temporalis muscles and right and left masseters (*bottom*) after one of the rewriting of the software. Green tracings: opening; red tracings: closing R right, L left.

1.3.5 2002: From K6-I to a customized and portable K7-I – the software is rewritten again

The K7-I is the latest and most evolved model in use today, particularly regarding hardware and EMG recording. It can be connected to a laptop via USB, and the K7-I itself can be moved (Figures 1.19, 1.22, and 1.23). The software for analyzing chewing cycles was yet again rewritten for the third time in accordance with the improved understanding of the clinical significance of chewing patterns acquired in the meantime.

Certainly, as time passed, and hundreds of chewing cycles from patients were rigorously classified, grouped, and recorded, we were able to identify from this mass of computer data the most significant figures from a clinical point of view. The last-generation program represents an important step forward, particularly in calculating the mean cycle and in EMG recording. Furthermore, the coordinates of points and angles of clinical significance are automatically provided in *diagnostic charts* to make it easier to interpret graphs and statistical analysis of results. The mean cycle and EMG activity are presented in linear graph form, whilst standard deviation is represented by an area chart. In the first program, standard deviation was displayed with horizontal lines, whilst in the new program an *area chart* is used to give a more realistic idea of the movement. This innovation is important, in that the standard deviation represents pattern variability, which is a physiological feature. The shape and position of the area represents diagnostic data which can be visually memorized more quickly and easy than lines (Piancino *et al.*, 2008) (Figures 1.20 and 1.21).

The instrument and program described (and currently in use) are for research purposes. Thanks to the results collected, a simple and quick system, utilizing wearable inertial units, is currently being developed to allow doctors to gather useful functional data for everyday use in their work.

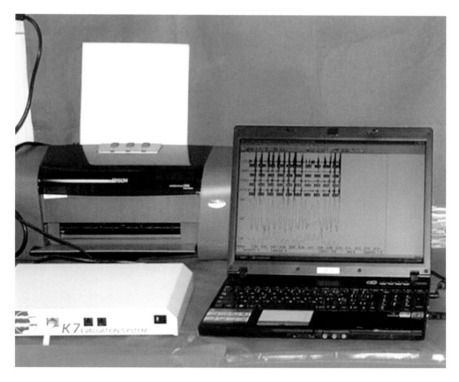

Figure 1.19   K7-I kinesiograph (Myotronics, Tukwila, WA, USA).

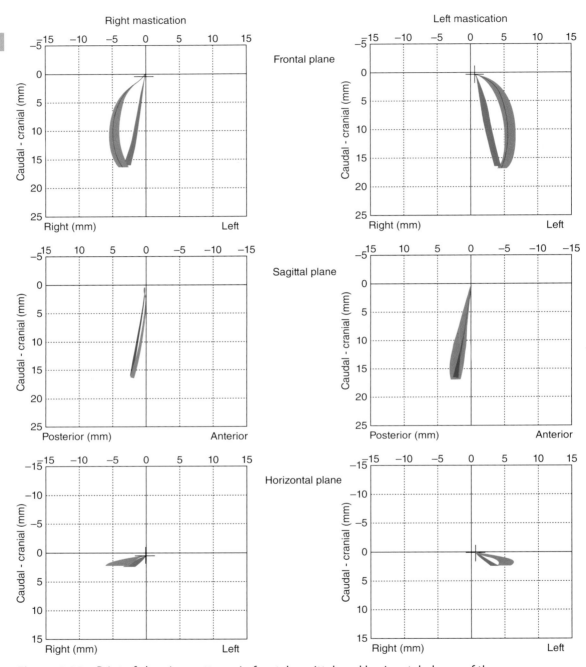

Figure 1.20 Print of chewing patterns in frontal, sagittal, and horizontal planes of the program dedicated to the K7-I kinesiograph; the solid line (green for the opening pattern and red for the closing pattern) represents the average chewing cycle of three trials lasting 10 s each. The green and red shaded areas represent the standard deviation from the average cycle.

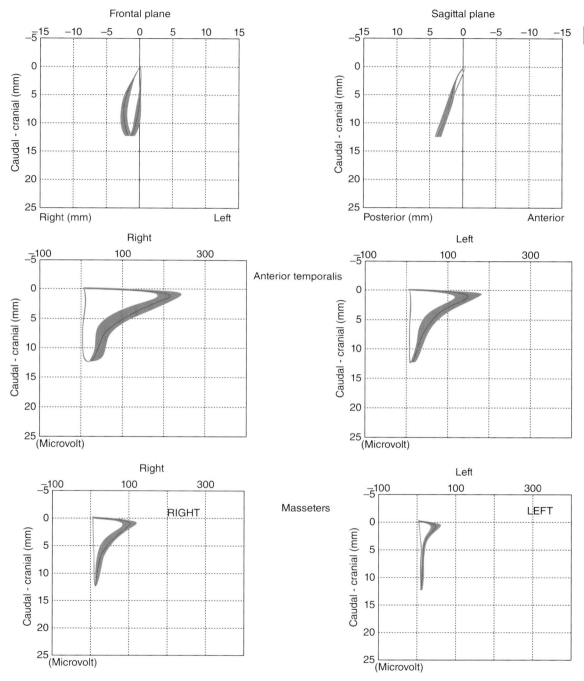

Figure 1.21 Print of an average chewing pattern in the frontal and sagittal planes (*top*); electromyography envelope plotted versus the vertical jaw displacement. The solid line (green for the opening pattern and red for the closing pattern) represents the average chewing cycle of three trials lasting 10 s each. The green and red shaded areas represent the standard deviation from the average cycle.

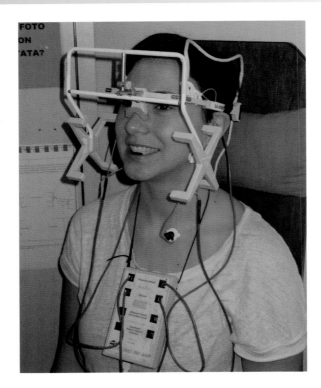

Figure 1.22   Multiple-sensor lightweight array of K7-I kinesiograph (Myotronics, Tukwila, WA, USA).

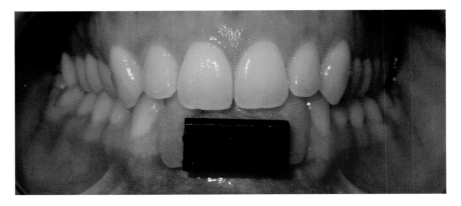

Figure 1.23   Magnet of the K7-I kinesiograph (Myotronics, Tukwila, WA, USA).

1.4 From the 1980s to today

1.4.1 The bolus

One of the most important aspects in a reliable study of masticatory function is surely *the choice and standardization of the bolus*. In fact, as stated in the literature (Lewin, 1985; Plesh *et al.*, 1986; Bishop *et al*, 1990; Shiau, 1999; Miyawaki *et al.*, 2000, 2001; Lassauzay *et al.*, 2000, Shiga *et al.*, 2001; Anderson *et al.*, 2002; Piancino *et al.*, 2008), the morphology of the pattern is directly linked to the chemical–physical characteristics of the bolus and its size. Random or varying choices of bolus types added to nonhomogeneous protocols, and sample selections means that masticatory research detailed in the literature is difficult to compare and standardize, and may even be unreliable at times.

The initial stages of research were carried out using simple chewing gum. From A. Lewin's work, it was clear that the use of both soft and hard bolus types in diagnosis was important to compare the patterns achieved and the capacity of the stomatognathic system to adapt to load (i.e., the differing bolus consistency). Thus, much attention was paid to the choice and standardization of bolus types; and from the very beginning, in the mid-1980s, patients with their own teeth were tested with two standardized boluses in terms of weight and dimension, according to parameters still adopted today: a soft bolus and a hard bolus. The soft bolus is a chewing gum, first softened up by the patient. The chewing cycles achieved with this bolus represent an "ideal" mastication as it does not change in consistency or volume and offers only limited resistance, thus submitting the system to low load. The hard bolus, on the other hand, is a winegum that does not stick to the teeth, changes consistency and volume as it is chewed, and demonstrates the true masticatory capacity. Many tests were carried out to identify the best type of bolus to use in order to allow a comparison of exertion: both boluses were the same size (20 mm in length, 1.2 mm in height, and 0.5 mm in width) but of different weights (2 g for the soft bolus and 3 g for the hard bolus) and different consistency (puncture forces 0,36 N for the soft bolus and 1,85 N for the hard bolus). But it is the comparison of patterns achieved with two boluses (as opposed to an absolute evaluation of one bolus or another) that allows the diagnosis of "capacity to adapt to load," as Lewin defined it.

The standardization of bolus types (like the standardization of the protocol, the position of the patient, etc.) is essential in achieving reliable and repeatable tests. We would like to make it clear that, in order to be of diagnostic importance, the recording of mastication must have a "test of exertion" as opposed to just a spontaneous instinctive movement that is subject to unacceptable variables for any type of scientific research. In any case, knowing that mastication is influenced by the limbic system also, it is important to know and respect the patients' taste in order to choose the most suitable *flavor of the bolus* (e.g., spearmint or strawberry chewing gum). If a spearmint chewing gum is given to a patient who hates this taste, the chewing pattern recorded will be pathologically false and of no clinical significance.

The types of bolus described are suitable to the recording of chewing cycles in patients with their own teeth – they cannot be used for toothless individuals or with tools that require different duration of sets of chewing, which instead require specific bolus types expressly made.

1.4.2 The protocol

The instrument used in this type of research is a kinesiograph, which involves the insertion of a small *magnet to the labial surfaces of the mandibular incisors* alongside *a headframe* that consists of an antenna system (to record the changes of the magnetic field) in the manner of an eyeglass. The kinesiograph also records the aligned *EMG activity of four masticatory muscles*: the right and left temporalis muscles, and the right and left masseters. Earlier, we described the complex but essential progression from single kinematic recordings to the simultaneous acquisition of jaw movement and EMG activity. The choice of the kinesiograph tool was not accidental, as may initially appear, but was the result of long deliberation by bioengineers. The alternative was an optoelectronic device. The kinesiograph was chosen instead because it was easier to use and provided more reliable results, important factors in large-scale clinical testing where a lot of data are lost during the process.

The protocol for recording chewing cycles, like the choice of bolus, was refined in collaboration with Lewin after long and careful experimentation. Indeed, *the protocol and bolus choices remain the same to this day* and produce diagnostic data that is both suitable and necessary for a complete diagnosis both of mandibular movement and of the related neuromuscular activity. The key factors are:

1. *The position of the patient during the test.* This is vital in achieving reliable and repeatable results. Thus, the position of the patient must not be casual but needs to be standardized – seated upright, legs at 90° and eyes fixed on a point 1 m away. This position is designed to reduce indirect movement to a minimum, (i.e. those movements related to mastication, particularly of the neck), in order to record mandibular movement connected to bolus chewing as precisely as possible. We know from the literature that the neck muscles and masticatory muscles mutually coordinate, and that holding the head steady allows indirect movement of the mandible to be prevented (Eriksson *et al.*, 1998).

2. *The test protocol.* The test involves deliberate mastication on the right side and on the left side, and free mastication. Each masticatory set is repeated three times, first with a soft bolus and then with a hard one. In total, nine sets with soft bolus and nine sets with hard bolus are recorded. Each set lasts 10 s, the mean time of mastication before swallowing occurs (Piancino *et al.*, 2008) (Figure 1.24).

3. *The recording of EMG activity.* As already mentioned, the recording of muscle activation requires the acquisition via surface electrodes of four of the eight masticatory muscles (i.e. the frontal temporalis muscles and the masseters). For anatomical reasons, the remaining four muscles (inner and outer medial and lateral pterygoids) are not compatible with the use of surface electrodes. However, if used correctly, the frontal temporalis and masseter muscles supply more than sufficient data for the purposes of understanding a patient's chewing conditions. Although modern technology would certainly allow it, it was decided not to expand the collection of data via surface electrodes to other muscles (such as the opening muscles or those of the neck) because, considering the clinical and statistical complexity of the masticatory system, it was preferred to concentrate on those masticatory muscles most directly involved in chewing. Over time, this was proven to be a wise decision, and currently it would be simple, if necessary, to expand EMG readings.

We wind up this topic by underlining that mastication is a complex function, the study of which requires considerable clinical experience, combined with appropriate instruments and protocols. Only in this way can reliable and clinically significant data be gathered.

1.5 Ready to start

Having described the clinical objectives, technological difficulties, and evolution of the research, as well as outlining the general characteristics of mastication and the study of this process, we are now ready to explore the topic more in depth. Chapters 2 and 3 are dedicated to the physiology of mastication, which is an essential factor in understanding the functional anomalies connected to malocclusion, or conditions of pain and dysfunction, and so on. As stated in the title, this book is dedicated to one type of malocclusion in particular: *the unilateral crossbite,*

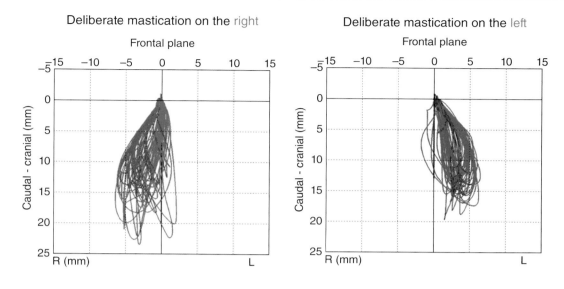

Deliberate mastication on the right

Deliberate mastication on the left

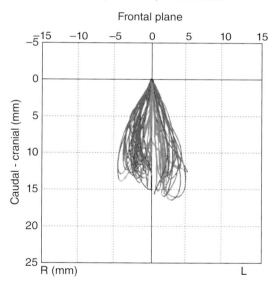

Free (alternate) mastication

Figure 1.24 Print of the superimposed chewing cycles in the frontal plane: deliberate right-hand and left-hand mastication (*top*); free (alternate) mastication (*bottom*). Green tracings: opening; red tracings: closing.

the form most responsible for altering physiological mastication (Figures 1.25 and 1.26). This condition is more serious the earlier it occurs, worsening over time, and irreversible once skeletal maturity has been reached. The task was to refine a therapeutic treatment suitable for the correction and prevention of such a disabling condition of the stomatognathic system. At the same time, an effort was made to understand the changes to masticatory function that are directly linked to unilateral crossbite, and to check that the treatment not only corrected the

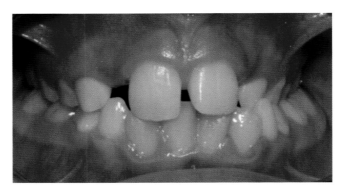

Figure 1.25   Left unilateral posterior crossbite before correction in mixed dentition.

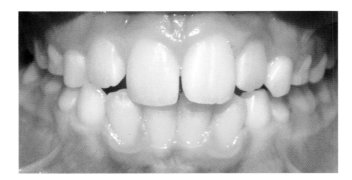

Figure 1.26   Dental occlusion after functional correction.

malocclusion but also restored the functional capacity. *This book will cover this issue, hopefully in a manner as clear and unquestionable as the results of tests in this field themselves.* Many other results linked to other types of malocclusion, neurological conditions, orthopedic conditions, prosthetic rehabilitation, and so on we have also been gathered, verified, and published, but, given the complexity and current scarcity of literature on this topic, we have chosen to limit the extent of this book as an introductory work in order to allow the reader to focus on, and understand more easily, the results of this study.

References

Ahlgren, J. (1967) Pattern of chewing and malocclusion of teeth. A clinical study. *Acta Odontol Scand* 25(1), 3–13.

Anderson K, Throckmorton GS, Buschang PH, Hayasaki H. (2002) The effects of bolus hardness on masticatory kinematics. *J Oral Rehabil* 29, 689–696.

Bernier AP, Arsenault I, Lund JP, Kolta A. (2010) Effect of the stimulation of sensory inputs on the firing of neurons of the trigeminal main sensory nucleus in the rat. *J Neurophysiol* 103(2), 915–923.

Bishop B, Plesh O, McCall WD. (1990) Effects of chewing frequency and bolus hardness on human incisor trajectory and masseter muscle activity. *Arch Oral Biol* 35, 311–318.

Bracco P, Viora E, Deregibus A, Piancino MG. (1990) Presentazione dell'hardware e del software dell'ultima generazione per l'elaborazione dei dati sirognatografici ed elettromiografici. *Riv It Stom* 7–8, 27–34.

Bracco P, Anastasi G, Maria Grazia Piancino MG, *et al.* (2010). Hemispheric prevalence during chewing in normal right-handed and left-handed subjects: a functional magnetic resonance imaging preliminary study. *Cranio* 28, 114–121.

Bracco P, Piancino MG, Talpone F, *et al.* (1999) Presentazione e spiegazione delle griglie numeriche per l'interpretazione diagnostica dei cicli masticatori. *Min Ortognat* 17, 25–33.

Dellow PG, Lund JP (1971) Evidence for central timing of rhythmical mastication. *J Physiol* 215(1), 1–13.

Eriksson P-O, Zafar H, Nordh E. (1998) Concomitant mandibular and head–neck movements during jaw opening–closing in man. *J Oral Rehabil* 25, 859–870.

Ferrario VF, Sforza C. (1996) Coordinated electromyographic activity of the human masseter and temporalis anterior muscles during mastication. *Eur J Oral Sci* 104, 511–517.

Kawamura Y. (1974) *Physiology of mastication.* Frontiers of oral physiology, vol. 1. Karger, Basel, pp. 121–158.

Lassauzay C, Peyron MA, Albuisson E, *et al.* (2000) Variability of the masticatory process during chewing of elastic model foods. *Eur J Oral Sci* 108, 484–492.

Lewin A. (1985) *Electrognathographics. An atlas for diagnostic procedures and interpretation.* Quintessence, Berlin.

Lundeen HC, Gibbs CH (1982) *Advances in occlusion.* J. Wright–PSG, Boston, MA.

Miyawaki S, Ohkochi N, Kawakami T, Sugimura M. (2000) Effect of food size on the movements of the mandibular first molars and condyles during deliberate unilateral mastication in humans. *J Dent Res* 79, 1525–1531.

Miyawaki S, Ohkochi N, Kawakami T, Sugimura M. (2001) Changes in masticatory muscle activity according to food size in experimental human mastication. *J Oral Rehabil* 28, 778–784.

Moller E. (1966) The chewing apparatus. An electromyographic study of the action of the muscles of mastication and its correlation to facial morphology. *Acta Physiol Scand* 280, 1–229.

Nakamura Y, Sessle GJ (1990) *Neurobiology of mastication. From molecular to system approach.* Elsevier, Tokyo, pp. 504–514.

Neff P. (1999) *TMJ occlusion and function.* Georgetown University School of Dentistry, Washington, DC. http://peterneffdds.com/blog, http://www.amazon.com/TMJ-occlusion-function-Peter-Neff/dp/B0006RE5SK (accessed October 2, 2015).

Plesh O, Bishop B, McCall WD. (1986) Effects of gum hardness on chewing pattern. *Exp Neurol* 92, 502–512.

Piancino MG, Bracco P, Vallelonga T, *et al.* (2008) Effect of bolus hardness on the chewing pattern and activation of masticatory muscles in subjects with normal dental occlusion. *J Electromyogr Kinesiol* 18(6), 931–937.

Purves D, Augustine GJ, Fitzpatrick, *et al.* (2000) *Neuroscienze* (trans. RLucchi, APoli, MVirgili). Zanichelli, Bologna.

Shiau YY, Peng CC, Hsu CW. (1999) Evaluation of biting performance with standardized test-foods. *J Oral Rehabil* 26, 447–452.

Shiga H, Stohler C, Kobayashi Y. (2001) The effect of bolus size on the chewing cycle in human. *Odontology* 89, 49–53.

Takada K, Nagata M, Miyawaki S, *et al.* (1992) Automatic detection and measurement of EMG silent periods in masticatory muscles during chewing in man. *Electromyogr Clin Neurophysiol* 32, 499–505.

Witter DJ, Woda A, Bronkhorst EM, Creugers NH. (2013) Clinical interpretation of a masticatory normative indicator analysis of masticatory function in subjects with different occlusal and prosthodontics status. *J Dent* 41(5), 443–448.

Woda A. (1984) *Fisiologia del sistema stomatognatico.* Elsevier–Masson, Milan.

Chapter 2

Physiology of Mastication: The Chewing Pattern and Masticatory Function

Contents

Understanding Masticatory Function in Unilateral Crossbites, First Edition. Maria Grazia Piancino and Stephanos Kyrkanides.
© 2016 John Wiley & Sons, Inc. Published 2016 by John Wiley & Sons, Inc.

2.1 Introduction

Physiology of mastication is subdivided into two parts: the first, discussed in this chapter, is dedicated to the description of the chewing pattern; the second, in Chapter 3, is dedicated to the description of neuromuscular control. This is a didactic subdivision, of course, because they happen simultaneously. Before studying the chewing pattern (i.e. the kinetics of the mandible during chewing), we would like to describe the characteristics of the general features of the masticatory function. This is very important for understanding the results of the research from a clinical point of view.

2.2 Features of masticatory function

Mastication is a complex process, and its proper functioning is fundamental for a good quality of life during all its stages (childhood, adulthood, and old age). It is one of the most important functional movements of the stomatognathic system and is *a highly coordinated neuromuscular motor function* that is carried out thanks to quick mandibular movements *with continual adjustment of applied force*. The entire nervous system, peripheral receptors (responsible for sensory input), and masticatory muscles (through which brain response and adjustment of movement are controlled) are all continually involved during mastication.

It is a *functional, rhythmic and semi-automatic movement*. First, it is important to outline and analyze these three characteristics of masticatory function before describing the actual pattern itself, thus allowing the reader to approach the subject from a broader viewpoint. Indeed, understanding chewing patterns (in the sense of electrognathographic readings) is certainly an important aspect, but in order to understand masticatory function from a clinical–diagnostic–therapeutic point of view, it is much more important to consider the *wider question of kinematic and muscular coordination between the two sides of the dental arches*. This issue embodies the complexity of the topic, but it also offers an opportunity to understand the importance of the function of mastication, and hopefully to identify appropriate physiological treatments, particularly for infancy and adolescence (when physical development is still taking place).

2.2.1 Functional (Figure 2.1)

Mastication in humans is a functional movement that is phylogenetically ancient and characterized by a high level of precise neuromuscular motor control and programming:

2.2.1.1 Phylogenetically ancient

Phylogenesis is the study of evolution, of a series of transformations and development taking place in vegetal and animal organisms over centuries. Masticatory function is one of the oldest phylogenetic functional movements. Ontogenesis is the series of processes taking pace during the biological development of an organism, from the embryo to the organism's mature form. It is distinct from phylogenensis which refers to the evolutionary history of a species. During ontogenesis, the structure follows to the functional compensation and vice versa (Slavicek, 2002). *One example of structural asymmetry and disturbance following functional compensation is undoubtedly unilateral posterior crossbite (positional asymmetry or functional crossbite)*, which may develop in early infancy in deciduous dentition. The growth of one or more occluded teeth cusp to cusp or inverted on one side only of the dental arch, results in an asymmetric compensation of masticatory function. As a result, functional and muscular asymmetry will be followed by an asymmetric growth of the structures and resulting discordant development.

Characteristics of masticatory function

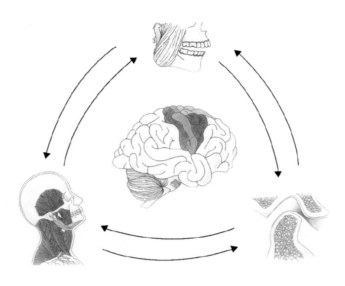

FUNCTIONAL	RHYTHMIC	SEMI-AUTOMATIC
- Phylogenetically ancient	- It is not a border movement	- Motor memory
- High neuromuscular control	- Simultaneously variable and repetitive	- Automatisms of neuromuscular control
- Precise motor control	- Bilateral coordination	- Adjustment to load

Figure 2.1 The masticatory system. The stomatognatic system: relationships between dental occlusion, TMJ, and neuromuscular control. *Source for the muscles:* Neff (1999). *Source for the brain:* Purves *et al.* (2000). Reproduced with the permission of Sinauer Associates.

2.2.1.2 *High level of neuromuscular control - an alternating movement*

Mastication may seem like a simple reflexive action, but it is in fact a complex function involving not only the entire stomatognathic system in a coordinated and precise process but also the *entire hierarchy of the central nervous system*, which is wired for motor cognitive sensory control (Takada and Myamoto, 2004; Hirano *et al.*, 2008). In humans, it is an alternating, rhythmic movement. Peripheral occlusal influences are fundamental in the establishment of chewing patterns: mechanoceptors and masticatory muscles show special, unusual features that allow them to adapt quickly and easily to the central demand and peripheral inputs as we will explain in chapter 3. Limbic issues and emotive characteristics of the patient also play a part in influencing certain features of chewing function (Bracco *et al.*, 2010).

2.2.1.3 *Precise motor control*

The programming of chewing action (as established by the central nervous system on the basis of peripheral input) is, as already mentioned, extremely precise and under continuous control. Thanks to this feature and continuous force adjustment, *the bolus is ground efficiently, avoiding harmful occlusal contact* that would quickly lead to serious damage and ruin of the stomatognathic system. *The peripheral receptors play an important role in this sense*, as they are highly concentrated and specialized within the stomatognathic system, and connected to the central nervous system. The messages sent to the central nervous system from this area are quick and detailed, and the muscles (by which the brain's reaction is received) allow an immediate and refined control of movement thanks to their particular anatomical features (macroscopic and microscopic). The need for motor control of chewing patterns is clear if one considers that the last part of closure (i.e., the stage near occlusion, dedicated to chewing of the bolus) has been likened to a ballistic-type movement. In fact, when dealing with high-precision trajectory, as maximum intercuspation is approached, the less controllable and modifiable does the mandibular movement become. *The precise neural control of the "occlusal phase of closing" is dedicated to the efficiency of grinding and the avoidance of traumatic injury and nociceptive stimuli from the teeth, in order to preserve and protect the stomatognathic system.* The concept of adjustment and compensation should be viewed in this context, and will be considered in Section 2.2.3.3.

2.2.2 **Rhythmic** (Figure 2.1)

Mastication is a *rhythmic action* that is performed with different mandibular patterns, established on the basis of peripheral information from the cortex, and maintained by the rhythmic pattern generator of the brainstem. Motor rhythm makes mastication unique amongst stomatognathic functions, particularly from the point of view of *neuromuscular motor control*. This is, in fact, characterized by precision and a remarkable *capacity for adjustment*. Variability and repetition are also intrinsic fundamental features, both of which are essential for correct physiological mastication even though they may seem to be contradictory characteristics.

Research shows that masticatory rhythm is maintained by the rhythmic pattern generator (situated in the pons and medulla oblongata of the brainstem) and some auto-firing cell groups in the nuclei at the base. The rhythmic patter generator of the brainstem is directly linked to neurons of Gasser's ganglion, transferring peripheral input from the stomatognathic receptors and, above all, from the periodontal mechano-receptors. These will be described in depth as they constitute the foundation of pattern programming and motor control of mastication. It seems apparently simple to understand how information arriving from the teeth is essential for establishing the chewing pattern (via cortical pathways) and controlling masticatory movement. We will look further at this topic later, but for now we want to highlight the importance of interaction between peripheral input and central network. *Rhythmic movement is thus a feature that needs rapid and precise neural control, and requires continual adjustment of the chewing pattern in order to protect the stomatognathic system and maintain maximum chewing efficiency.* To fully understand chewing patterns, the following features must be remembered:

2.2.2.1 *It is not a border movement*

The fact that mastication is not a border movement is important as we need to clarify from the outset the characteristics and differences of these two functional movements. *The border movements of the mandible are voluntary*, and of vital significance in the field of dentistry. They provide a reference point that is universally recognized and adopted from both diagnostic and therapeutic viewpoints, all over the world. They can be considered functional movements, but they are *voluntary and not rhythmic*. Mastication, on the other hand, is rhythmic and semi-automatic and involves mandibular and condylar displacement, which are very different from border movements. In the 1980s, gnathologists discovered to their surprise (Slavicek, 2002) that the condyle tracks recorded during border movements are different and not overlapping with those recorded during mastication. It is clear, then, that to avoid confusion, the importance of a specific and bespoke terminology is undeniable when talking about mastication.

From the field of medicine, we know the importance of appropriate terminology to prevent confusion caused by apparently similar diagnostic frameworks which are in fact different from both dynamic and clinical viewpoints. We believe a dedicated terminology is essential, as opposed to a derived terminology as often occurs in fields other than dentistry, because there remains a risk that imprecise and unsuitable terms be used, introducing biases and obscuring the clinical meaning of the results. This question will be further considered at the end of this chapter but, as a quick example, we can say that for a correct analysis of chewing patterns, we will refer to the "bolus side" (and not "working" side), as well as the "contralateral side of the bolus" as opposed to "balancing side").

2.2.2.2 *Variable and repeatable*

An important characteristic of masticatory pattern, as we have already mentioned, is the simultaneous presence of variability and repetitivity, co-existing within chewing patterns (Lewin, 1985). *Repetitivity* allows the detection of the chewing cycle pattern. An established chewing pattern is important for efficient grinding of the bolus and avoiding dental trauma. *Variability*, on the other hand, represents the freedom of mandibular movement (which is a sign of physiological wellbeing), muscles that are not overloaded, and articular *loads* that are *symmetrically and well distributed* (Lewin et al., 1995). Patterns that are totally repetitive (lacking freedom of movement and with overloading of the elements) are instead pathological conditions, as are patterns that are totally variable (lacking motor memory and patterns).

2.2.2.3 *Bilateral coordination and alternating movement*

At the beginning of this section we underlined that understanding masticatory pattern (in the sense of an electrognathographic reading) is, of course, essential, but we must also not forget to take a broader look at kinematic and muscular coordination between the two sides of the dental arches, if the study is to evolve in clinical and therapeutic terms.

We know, in fact, that *healthy mastication by humans consists of an "alternating" movement*. This vital characteristic underpins the symmetry of the movement, of the neuromuscular loading, and the structural/joint effort. The single chewing pattern supplies valid and useful input, but *the importance of bilateral evaluation* must never be neglected if one is to completely understand the *clinical significance of masticatory function*.

Bilateral coordination requires, of course, *bilateral neuromuscular control*. This means that we cannot look independently or definitively at the muscle either on the bolus side or on the contralateral side, as individual variability does not allow reliable results. But studying the relationship between the muscle on the bolus side and that on the contralateral side reveals reliable data that is both repeatable and of clinical interest. In this way, *the study of mastication is significantly different from the countless studies of teeth clenching*, which can be compared with the border movements previously described, but have nothing in common with mastication.

Bilateral coordination implies a remarkable complexity of mathematical–statistic calculations, which underpin this study. We have no intention whatsoever of boring our readers with this topic; we would just like to underline that in order to understand a complex and fundamental function such as mastication, and develop this topic from diagnostic and therapeutic viewpoints, then even though we set off with a look at specific considerations (regarding patterns), we must never lose view of the overall idea (bilateral coordination).

2.2.3 **Semi-automatic** (Figure 2.1)

The term *semi-automatic* movement is purely neurological and indicates a movement managed by automatisms in the nervous system (brainstem, cerebellum, basal nuclei, cortex) that is, however, voluntarily started and constantly controlled by the cerebral cortex. Thus, it can be interrupted or modified at will. This characteristic is shared by other physiological functions, such as breathing or walking.

2.2.3.1 Motor memory

A rhythmic movement like chewing is subject to precise and complex motor control, intended to protect the condition of the stomatognathic system, and involving "motor memory." On the basis of dental, structural, and articular characteristics, as well as bolus features (consistency, volume, etc.), all of which send data by peripheral receptors, the cerebral cortex sets the most suitable pattern that is then maintained by rhythm centers and continually adjusted by feedback and feed-forward automatic mechanisms.

Some precocious malocclusions, such as unilateral posterior crossbite, have a strong influence on the motor memory of masticatory function, establishing an anomalous pattern that is then deeply resistant to change (Throckmorton *et al.*, 2001).

2.2.3.2 Automatisms of neuromuscular control

The automatic mechanisms charged to the central nervous system's motor control are *genetically determined and inherited, and may alter as a result of use and experience*. They are complex mechanisms, dependent on the activity of the cerebral cortex, basal nuclei, cerebellum, and brainstem. They are considerably different from reflex actions, which are instead totally nonvoluntary and can be viewed as simpler movements. *The fine-tuning of automatisms and motor memory (starting with peripheral input) begins at birth, and any correction/modification/improvement to these requires time and, above all, appropriate treatment.*

It is important for all dentists and orthodontists to understand these features, especially for orthodontists who are called on to correct not only dental but also stomatognathic abnormalities in growing children. Understanding masticatory function is now essential in the diagnosis of orthodontic malocclusion, in order to identify the best treatment for dental and, above all, functional repair.

2.2.3.3 Adjustment and compensation (Figure 2.1)

At this point we would like to underline that Sections 2.2.1, 2.2.2, and 2.2.3, which generally describe masticatory function (as functional, rhythmic, and semi-automatic), are based on neurological control features; that is, the true base of mastication, which is strictly linked to occlusion and to the structures of the stomatognathic system. Without a firm understanding of the role of neurological control, it is impossible to understand mastication and its clinical effects. The subject is, however, easy to understand with a minimum amount of effort and a willingness to forget old, outdated concepts.

We now want to look at the frequently misunderstood feature of the *capacity for adjustment* in order to allow the reader to comprehend better the role of function. The ability of the stomatognathic system to adapt to change is remarkable and allows professionals in different fields to adopt a wide variety of therapeutic treatments. This is particularly important for dentists and orthodontists, who work on tissues as hard as teeth. So, obviously, *the capacity for adjustment is a physiological characteristic* of the system without which everyday life would be difficult. However, clinical experience and professional integrity are necessary to understand the fine line that is passed between *adjustment and compensation, knowing that the latter gives way to the likelihood of developing diseases/harmful conditions*. In order to protect the structures of the stomatognathic system and avoid harmful input, neural control establishes a functional compensation according to the structure, which in turn remodels itself according to its functional alteration (Slavicek, 2002; Kandel *et al.*, 2012). The system is complex – interactions between the structure and neural control are strictly linked, multiple and bi-unique, and therefore often difficult, if not impossible, to diagnose. The problem arises due to the fact that, in some cases, quite apart from adjustment that is related to physiological changes during physiological growing and aging, a real functional compensation is called for to respond to a structural endogenous pathology or traumatism or therapeutic side effects. In such an event, *the system is able to "compensate" the error but not to autocorrect.* If it is later accompanied by other "external or therapeutical trauma," other functional compensations will be activated without correcting again *the original error,* which *becomes an integral and conditioning feature from a structural and functional point of view.* Current diagnostic methods do not allow a precise diagnosis of exactly how, which and how many organs are involved by compensation. This is due to the complexity and *multifaceted character of the system.* Compensation can lead (over time and with the amounting of other errors or compensations from different locations) to chronic or acute pain that at the stage of its occurence, is very difficult to cure because, we repeat, it is a multifaceted and *multidisciplinary issue,* and because after a certain point the system has limited reaction capacity. In other words, the functional compensation may become a serious risk in a complex system. The only way to avoid this risk (and to "cure," in the medical sense of the word, young children still in the stages of orthodontic development and adults requiring orthodontic repair treatment), is *to achieve structural relationships both at the end but especially during all therapies that steadily allow the best physiological function possible.* For example, in this book we will explain how unilateral posterior crossbite causes or is caused by an alteration of the chewing pattern to compensate for malocclusion. The result of this malocclusion is a functional imbalance, identified statistically. This asymmetrical function is followed by an asymmetric remodeling of all the structures in the stomatognathic system – this remodeling is more intense in developing children, but it also occurs in adults. The system functionally compensates the occlusion error (i.e., the crossbite malocclusion), but is not able to correct the error. If appropriate treatment from a physiological point of view is adopted, in order to recover function, the system resets itself and thus all the structures grow together harmoniously. If, on the other hand, the malocclusion (the "error") is not corrected or is corrected with traumatic therapies requiring compensation in thier turn, the system will compensate by establishing an asymmetrical function after the occlusal asymmetry and the structures will consequently grow asymmetrically – in this way, all the errors becomes an integrated part of the system. Once fully developed, the dissymmetry will be both irreversible and incurable.

The search for the best functional balance during therapy may appear complex, but if one begins with the knowledge of the functions of the stomatognathic system and how to adopt the consistent therapeutic solutions, it becomes easy to comprehend and, above all, have the satisfaction of seeing and understanding the reasons for its rebalancing.

Dental and orthodontic therapies thus fulfill an important functional role linked to gnathological functions and the patient's quality of life. From this point of view we would like to underline *the role of the stomatognathic system in personal relationships, cognitive activity, stress management and quality of life.* Dentists are physicians involved in the "cure" of one of the most important system of the human body (Slavicek, 2002).

2.3 Terminology

As mentioned earlier, we now want to look at an issue that many still often find confusing – terminology. This is essential in order to understand and correctly interpret the clinical meaning of mastication. It is important to clearly establish (with precision and scientific reasoning) the correct terminology to use when speaking or writing about mastication. The incorrect use of a term is not just a simple mistake of form – it can lead to biases, misunderstandings, false readings, and mistaken diagnoses, all of which can be easily avoided.

Here, we list and then explain some of the terms used in this book:

- bolus side
- contralateral side to bolus side

- maximum functional intercuspation
- occlusal phase of closure
- muscular coordination
- adjustment to load
- chewing pattern
- reverse-sequence chewing cycles
- adjustment
- compensation
- sagittal condylar pattern.

The reader may also update the terminology of masticatory function using the page Appendix: Terminology update.

2.3.1 Bolus side

This is the side of the dental arch where the bolus is positioned and where grinding takes place. When talking about mastication, it is important to define which is the side of the bolus and which is the contralateral side. Unfortunately, some authors referring to mastication use the alternative terms "working side" (bolus side) and "balancing side" (contralateral side). This is however the terminology referring to the border movements of the mandible. As we will see, the characteristics of mastication are very different from those of border movements. So, it is vital to clearly distinguish between the two terminologies. Since the mandibular and condylar movements during grinding of the bolus are quite different from border movements, in this book we will always use the terms "bolus side" and "contralateral side".

2.3.2 Contralateral side to bolus side

This is the dental arch opposite the bolus side, with which it shares coordinated (but not grinding) movement. For the sake of simplicity, the term "contralateral to bolus side" can be shortened to simply "contralateral side."

2.3.3 Maximum functional intercuspation

When a bolus (especially a hard bolus) is held between the upper and lower teeth, the position of initial maximum static intercuspation cannot be achieved, but during mastication there are various points of maximum closure (the stage nearest maximum static intercuspation), in a continual state of flux until the bolus is completely shredded. These points have been defined as maximum functional intercuspation in order to indicate the nearest point of a determined chewing cycle to the initial maximum static intercuspation stage.

2.3.4 Occlusal phase of closure

The occlusal phase of closure refers to the final stage of closure, immediately prior to functional intercuspation. At this point when the force is expressed, the bite force involved in grinding the bolus and its trajectory are indicators of efficient chewing function (Wilding and Lewin, 1994). It has also been defined as the power phase of closure followed by the transcuspidal and intercuspidal phase of mastication (Lewin, 1985).

2.3.5 Muscular coordination

This term is a generic definition that takes on a particular meaning in the context of mastication – in this field, the EMG amplitude (i.e., muscular activation in its absolute sense) has little or no clinical significance because the level of individual variability and the factors influencing this are significant and mean that any clinical results should be viewed as questionable. On the other hand, the evaluation of coordination between muscles on the two sides (bolus and contralateral) or between different types of masticatory muscles is of fundamental importance and generally reliable. All evaluations of muscular activity during mastication are based on the principle of "muscular coordination," which is maintained and protected even in the case of malocclusion.

2.3.6 Adjustment to load

Once again, despite appearing generic, this concept is in fact of primary importance in the study of mastication. The ability of the stomatognathic system to "adjust to load," both from kinematic and muscular points of view, is a physiological characteristic that operates as an indicator in the diagnosis of physiological masticatory function.

2.3.7 Chewing pattern (Figure 2.2)

The chewing pattern is made up of an average of single chewing cycles and displays a personal characteristic morphology for each patient. It is never the same, being in a constant flux according to a precise motor program memorized in the central nervous system. Absence of a pattern (i.e., the total irregularity of chewing cycles) indicates a serious malfunction in the masticatory system.

2.3.8 Reverse-sequencing chewing cycle

A reverse-sequence chewing cycle is one in which the closing vector in the final stage of the closure pattern has a reverse sequence to the norm. In other words, cycles characterized by clockwise closure in normal physiological conditions demonstrate anti-clockwise closure, and vice versa when they are reversed. A single, or few, reverse-sequence cycles are not pathognomonic and have no clinical significance. What is important is the percentage number of reverse cycles compared with the overall total number of cycles completed.

2.3.9 Adjustment

This is the ability of the neuromuscular system to adapt its function to physiological changes occurring in physiological conditions in humans during growing and over time.

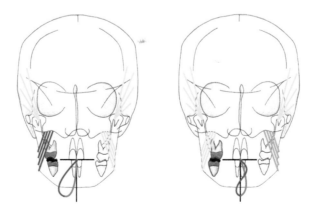

Physiological mastication
Right-hand side

Reverse sequence mastication
Right-hand side

Figure 2.2 Physiological versus reverse chewing cycle. Green tracings: opening; red tracings: closing.

2.3.10 Compensation

This is the ability of the neuromuscular system to change function due to structural pathologies (endogenous or traumatic), nonphysiological therapies, external agents, and so on. Unlike
adjustment that is related to physiological aging, compensation can be viewed as a reaction to
a pathological situation, which may, in turn, cause other worsening pathologies.

2.3.11 Sagittal condylar pattern

This is the path of the condyle on either the bolus or contralateral side during mastication.
Knowing that they are different between sides, the definition "sagittal condylar pattern" is
incomplete and needs to be rendered more precise with the addition of "bolus side" or "contralateral." It is significantly different from the sagittal condylar path recorded by an axiograph,
which belongs in the terminology of border movements, as it differs physiologically between
the two sides.

2.3.12 Acronyms used in this book

Few acronyms have been used in this book, in order to facilitate reading. The acronyms used are
usually well-known and are the following:

electromyography = EMG
tamporo-mandibular joint = TMJ
central nervous system = SNC
sarcoglicans = SCG
function generating bite appliance = FGB

2.4 The chewing pattern

So far, we have described the general characteristics of mastication – the rhythm, the
semi-automatic neuromuscular control, the symmetry between the sides, and balanced load
(Figure 2.3).

Bearing these aspects in mind, we will now begin to describe the features of chewing
patterns, in the sense of mandibular kinetics in opening and closure. Gibbs describes chewing

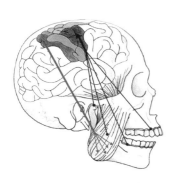
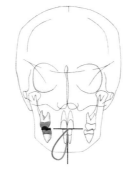
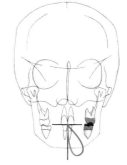

Mastication on the RIGHT   Mastication on the LEFT

Figure 2.3   Motor control and peripheral inputs during masticatory function.

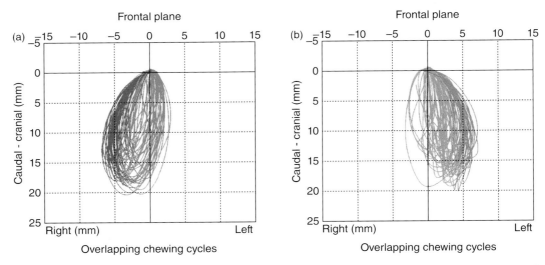

Figure 2.4 Overlapping chewing cycles in the frontal plane during chewing deliberately on the right (a) and left (b) side. Green tracings: opening; red tracings: closing.

patterns in interincisor, molar, and condylar levels, whilst Lewin offers his fundamental clinical interpretation of chewing patterns on an interincisor level (Lundeen and Gibbs, 1982; Lewin, 1985). The study of chewing patterns, if distanced from the general characteristics of mastication described so far, risks leading to sectorial and meaningless diagnoses. We need reliable and repeatable points of reference for chewing cycles, which will be described in this chapter, but the study of chewing patterns should never be detached from its context; that is, from the diagnostic data connected to occlusion, cephalometric and postural characteristics. Furthermore, *a bilateral (as opposed to unilateral) study of the pattern is of great clinical importance* (Figure 2.4). We hope that these concepts on which is based the whole book, will be clear for scientific referees and editors too, in order to stop unsuitable comments blocking the publications of important and reliable studies of interest for the clinical and scientific communities.

In the following section we will describe the results of research by Gibbs *et al.* (1981a–c, 1982), which we believe has made an essential contribution to explaining the bilateral characteristics of masticatory movement. The second part is dedicated to a skilled clinical interpretation of chewing pattern registered at the interincisive point according to Lewin, (thus referring to the two authors who have guided the research on which this book is based).

2.4.1 **First molar pattern** (Figures 2.5, 2.6, and 2.7)

This section examines the main findings on mastication by Gibbs and coworkers (Gibbs *et al.*, 1981a; Lundeen and Gibbs, 1982). We have already looked at the device used (the case gnathic replicator), which, despite being complex to use because of its heavy and unwieldy properties, had the advantage of being able to reliably and precisely track chewing cycles in humans for the first time. This tracking not only involved the interincisor level but also bilateral first molars and bilateral temporomandibular movement on the bolus and contralateral sides.

The results of the study into molar movement on the bolus and contralateral sides during mastication are surprising, as the two molars and condyles register different movements despite belonging to the same rigid skeletal structure.

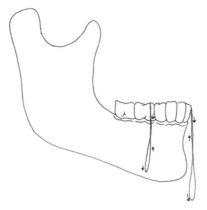

Figure 2.5   Kinetics of the right first molar, on the bolus side – sagittal plane. *Source:* Redrawn from Lundeen and Gibbs (1982). Reproduced with permission from Elsevier.

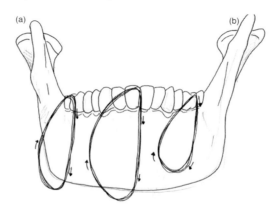

Figure 2.6   Kinetics of the mandible during chewing on the right side – frontal plane. Central tracing: recording at the incisal point; (a) recording at the first molar point on the bolus side; (b) recording at the first molar point on the contralateral side. *Source:* Redrawn from Lundeen and Gibbs (1982). Reproduced with permission from Elsevier.

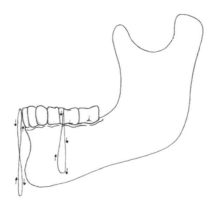

Figure 2.7   Kinetics of the left first molar on the contralateral chewing side – sagittal plane. *Source:* Redrawn from Lundeen and Gibbs (1982). Reproduced with permission from Elsevier.

2.4.1.1 First molar on bolus side

- *Opening:* during the opening phase, the molar on the bolus side moves forward and downward on the sagittal plane, whilst it shifts sideways on the bolus side on the frontal plane.
- *Closure:* in the occlusal phase of closure having retreated upwards, the molar moves forward and downward on the sagittal plane and medially on the frontal plane.

2.4.1.2 First molar on the contralateral side

- *Opening:* in the opening phase, the contralateral molar moves forward and downward on the sagittal plane, but medially on the frontal plane.
- *Closure:* in the occlusal phase of closure the molar shifts on the sagittal plane from an anterior and medial position in a backward and upward direction, whilst on the frontal plane it moves laterally.

2.4.1.3 Summary

The first molars on the bolus and contralateral sides follow different paths that do not coincide or overlap. As we will see, the patterns of the first molars are similar to the paths of their respective condyles. To obtain a symmetrical function, the alternate movement is important.

2.4.2 Condylar pattern in the frontal plane (Figures 2.8, 2.9, and 2.10)

2.4.2.1 Condyle of the bolus side

- *Opening:* during opening, the condyle on the bolus side moves forward and downward on the sagittal plane and laterally towards the bolus side on the frontal plane.
- *Closing phase I:* in the closure phase, the condyle on the bolus side moves upward and backward on the sagittal plane and laterally on the frontal plane.

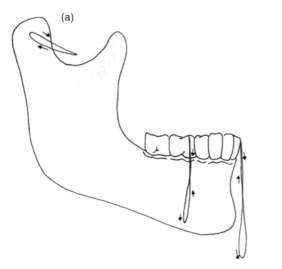 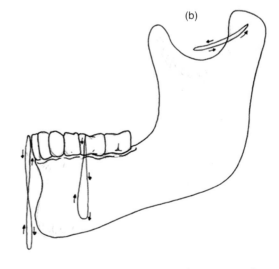

Figure 2.8 Kinetics of the right (a) bolus side and left (b) contralateral condyle during chewing on the right side – sagittal plane. Sagittal condylar tracings follow different trajectories. *Source:* Redrawn from Lundeen and Gibbs (1982). Reproduced with permission from Elsevier.

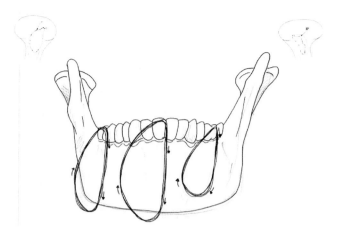

Figure 2.9   Kinetics of the mandible and condyles during chewing on the right side – frontal plane. The condylar patterns are different between sides. *Source:* Redrawn from Lundeen and Gibbs (1982). Reproduced with permission from Elsevier.

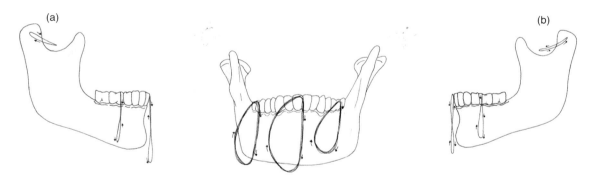

Figure 2.10   Kinetics of the condyles in the sagittal plane (a: bolus side; b: contralateral side) and in the frontal plane (center of the image). Opening and closing tracing follow different trajectories. *Source:* Redrawn from Lundeen and Gibbs (1982). Reproduced with permission from Elsevier.

- *Closing phase II:* the condyle moves forward (0.33 mm) downward and medially on the frontal plane (0.18 mm).
- On the sagittal plane, the opening and closing paths of the condyle on the bolus side do *not* overlap, and the opening phase registers a wider path than the closure.

2.4.2.2 Contralateral condyle on the bolus side

- *Opening:* during opening, the contralateral condyle on the bolus side moves forward and downward on the sagittal plane and medially on the frontal plane.

- *Closure:* during closure, the contralateral condyle moves backward and upward on the sagittal plane and laterally on the frontal plane, until it reaches its final position together with the teeth.
- On the sagittal plane, the opening and closing paths of the contralateral condyle are overlapping.

2.4.2.3 Summary

The condyle of the *bolus side* on the sagittal plane has *non-overlapping* opening and closing paths, as the opening path is higher than the closure.

The *contralateral* condyle on the sagittal plane has *overlapping* opening and closing paths.

Thus, during mastication there is no terminal hinge axis movement, and the TMJ load on the bolus side is different from that on the contralateral side.

This finding was confirmed by Naeije and Hofman (2003), when they concluded their article by hypothesizing that the load of the TMJ on the bolus side is less than that on the contralateral side. This would explain why some patients with unilateral TMJ dysfunction instinctively choose to chew on the side of the dysfunction because it is less loaded (Naeije and Hofman, 2003).

2.4.3 Condylar pattern in the sagittal plane during chewing in deciduous and permanent dentition (Figures 2.11 and 2.12)

During mastication, the incline of the sagittal condylar pattern in an adult is very different from that of a child with deciduous dentition. In fact, we know from Gibbs that the *sagittal condylar pattern* during mastication for a child with milk teeth presents an incline of approximately 15° compared with the horizontal axis, whereas *an adult* with permanent teeth presents *a sagittal condylar pattern* with an incline of *approximately 45°* compared with the horizontal axis, i.e. around half the value between the horizontal and vertical axes (Lundeen and Gibbs, 1982).

Such a significant difference in sagittal condylar patterns is related to variances in anatomical features, which, in turn, are related to the functional requirements of each period of life/age of the patient. In fact, at birth, TMJ movement is undeveloped and accompanied by a barely emerged condyle, an almost inexistent glenoid cavity, and an articular prominence that is still almost flat. The condyle is, in fact, one of the least developed joints at birth. Far from being coincidental, this anatomic characteristic thus allows forward and backward mandibular excursions on the sagittal plane, which is necessary for sucking action, an essential vital reflex.

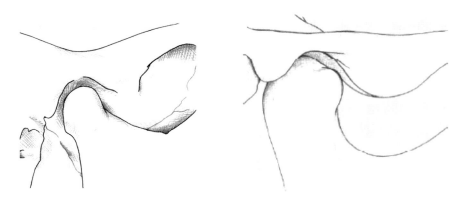

Figure 2.11   TMJ of a child with deciduous dentition (*left*) and of an adult with permanent dentition (*right*).

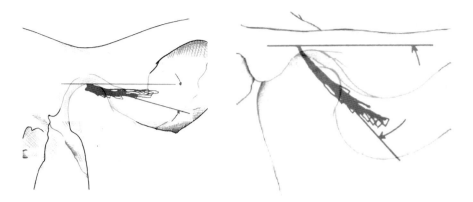

Figure 2.12   Sagittal condylar patterns during mastication in deciduous (*left*) and permanent (*right*) dentition.

At this point, the question arises: "How do these vital anatomical developments and changes in the TMJ take place?" From literature regarding clinical studies, *we know that the development of the TMJ has been defined as an "adaptive growth" type* (Ingervall *et al.*, 1976; Thilander *et al.*, 1976; Thilander, 2000). Almost all the development of the TMJ takes place after birth, *"adapting" itself to the postural, skeletal, occlusal, and neuromuscular features of the individual*, in close connection with the function of sucking at birth, and later of chewing (Katsavrias and Dibbets, 2001). The development of the TMJ and the resulting change in incline of the pattern on the sagittal plane are influenced by the adaptation of the structure to the changes in function.

With their occlusal contact and via mechanoreceptors, the teeth acquire a primary role in the neural establishment and control of masticatory function, which in turn affects skeletal and articular development. They can significantly contribute to righting the entire stomatognathic system, but conversely (in pathological cases or in cases of erroneous therapies) they can also cause a functional imbalance of the system and consequent incorrect structural adaptation. For this reason, an in-depth knowledge of the functioning of the stomatognathic system is essential for both orthodontists and prosthodontists – the former because they can re-establish healthy masticatory function in childhood and thus attune the growth of the entire system, and the latter because, by replacing lost teeth, they can restore neuromuscular and joint harmony of patients. This is the true goal of dental treatment and intervention.

2.5 The chewing pattern as an indicator of masticatory function

One of the most important contributions in literature to the clinical understanding of chewing patterns was undoubtedly made by A. Lewin, who, as explained earlier, used the Sirognatograph to record chewing cycles (Lewin, 1985). As already stated, this device allowed *the tracking of movement at just one point of the mandible* – the interincisive point. This method of tracking movement is still used today, although it has been considerably improved from a technical point of view as it now allows the acquisition of a large number of patients' readings in a simple and repeatable manner.

One of the aims of this book is to describe chewing patterns from the point of view of neuromuscular equilibrium and masticatory efficiency, identifying clinically significant features. First, however, we believe it important to emphasize that the analysis of chewing cycles described in this book is not a subjective interpretation but it is based on significant statistic results after

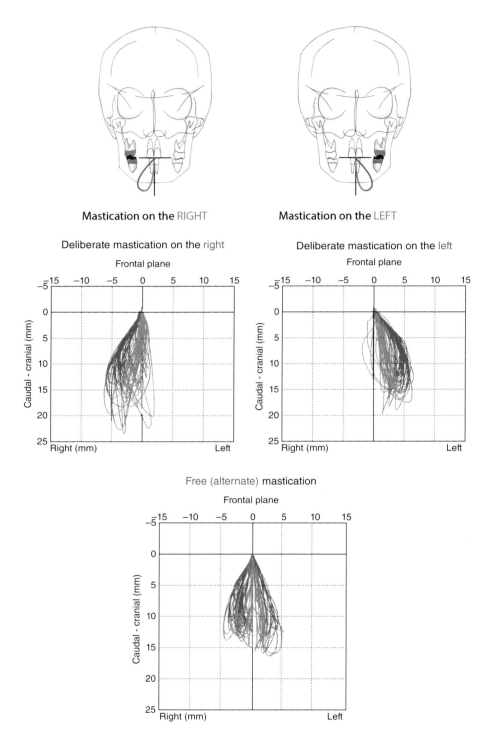

Figure 2.13 The physiological chewing pattern during chewing deliberately on the right and on the left side (*top*) and during free-alternate mastication (*bottom*). Green tracings: opening; red tracings: closing.

long years of research aimed at understanding which, and how many, of the "numeric data" supplied so easily by the devices may in fact be of clinical relevance.

The starting point was the high number of subjects categorized according to analyzed occlusal and cephalometric diagnostic data (recorded before and after orthodontic treatment). In view of the variability of the function, *all the results referred to here have been reconfirmed by different professionals on different groups of patients*. If the identified feature is valid and reliable, then results may be easily reconfirmed. We were asked, about 20 years ago, to write a textbook on chewing cycles, but at that time we refused because of insufficient data and lack of confirmed results. Today, we believe it is time to publish the reliable and repeatable results acquired, and this is why we have produced this book, which, as we said before, is not based on "opinions" but on solid and meaningful statistics. Of course, there is still much to discover, as masticatory function is connected to many other factors quite apart from the stomatognathic system, but the *understanding of dental influence on chewing patterns is a fundamental starting point*, without which it would be impossible for anyone to understand mastication or open up new multidisciplinary fields of study.

Thus, we can begin to seriously look at this issue by describing chewing patterns in general and then analyzing the various aspects point by point. This will give us an overall idea of mandibular movement, which is the final result and aim of the function. In Chapter 3 we will look at the neuromuscular system, a true protagonist in masticatory function and the result of integrated peripheral sensory input from motor programming, which involves the entire central nervous system, including the limbic nervous system.

A chewing pattern comprises two phases: the *opening pattern* (represented in this book in green), and the *closing pattern* (here represented in red). In conditions of physiological occlusion and healthy masticatory function, the pattern recorded at the lower interincisive point features:

• opening along the vertical axis;
• lateral movement on the bolus side in the last phase of opening and in the first stage of closure;
• medial movement of the occlusal phase of closure until functional intercuspation is reached.

2.5.1 **Symmetry and alternating movement** (Figure 2.13)

As mastication is a rhythmic and alternating movement, the morphology of a chewing cycle is a "semi-loop" during mastication on one side, as the other half of the "loop" occurs during mastication on the other side. In fact, during mastication of a bolus on the right-hand side, chewing cycles are developed on the right-hand side of the patient. Conversely, during mastication of a bolus on the left-hand side, the chewing patterns take place on the patient's left-hand side in a mirrored and symmetric manner. If we consider the left- and right-hand side chewing patterns together as a whole, the overall effect is that of a true "loop"-like shape. In normal healthy mastication, spontaneous chewing is an alternating-style movement, and chewing patterns with a right-side bolus are numerically balanced and symmetrical to those with a left-side bolus, albeit not identical.

The concept of *symmetry in normal chewing patterns* is extremely important because it indicates balance, good health and growth, and wellbeing of the stomatognathic system. When masticatory movement is alternate, mirrored, and symmetrical, the stomatognathic structures are rhythmically involved and able to exercise maximum force homogeneously distributed, avoiding harmful overloading of some parts of the system. The intrinsic alternance between sides is the basis of the symmetry of the movement. *Some occlusal conditions*, some functional malocclusions (which we will describe in Chapter 4) will *alter this symmetry of movement, creating a serious imbalance and gradually aggravated functional problems* with consequences for the dentoalveolar and cranial structures, especially in the period of infancy and childhood growth (Thilander *et al.*, 1976; Ronnerman and Thilander, 1978; Nerder *et al.*, 1999; Pinto *et al.*, 2001; Thilander and Lennartsson, 2002; Thilander *et al.*, 2002; Piancino *et al.*, 2009).

2.5.2 Repetitivity and variability (Figure 2.14)

We have already mentioned the importance of variability and repetitivity as features of masticatory function. These two concepts may seem contradictory, but the harmonious balance of both elements together is what characterizes healthy mastication. If one prevails over the other, however, this is an indication of some masticatory abnormality.

Repetitivity of the chewing cycle constitutes a chewing pattern and it requires rhythm, well-defined motor programming, firm dental contact, and ballistic-type movement. If repetitivity is absent, the chewing cycle becomes completely haphazard, lacking in motor programming and highly inefficient. This may happen, for example, immediately after orthognathodontic surgery, following a sudden change in peripheral input (Lewin, 1985; Ferrario *et al.*, 2006).

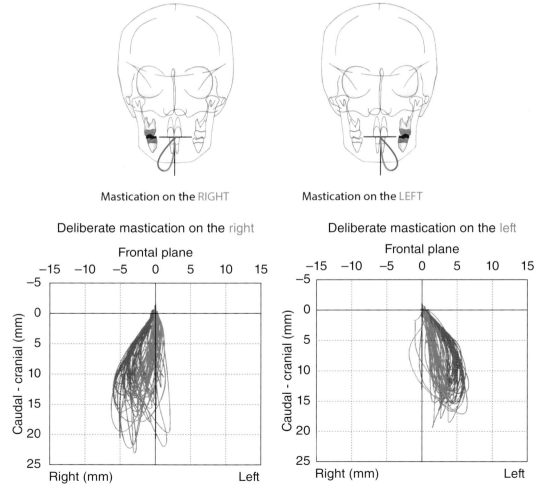

Figure 2.14 Overlapping chewing cycles during chewing deliberately on the right and on the left side, showing the repeatability and variability of the masticatory movement. Green tracings: opening; red tracings: closing.

Repetitivity is flanked by *variability of the chewing cycle*, which is never the same. The presence of variability indicates freedom of movement, healthy functioning, and appropriate load applied to muscles. If variability is absent, there will be a serious lack of freedom for mandibular movement, a freedom that is essential to avoid both neuromuscular overload with resulting muscle fatigue and the overloading of some areas of the TMJ with resulting alterations to anatomical structures and synovial fluid (Nitzan 2002, 2003; Nitzan and Etsion, 2002; Nitzan *et al.*, 2004). Pathologies that "imprison" the mandible in an enforced position in an attempt to avoid harmful contact to the stomatognathic system may often cause the aforesaid consequences. One example of such pathologies could be severe deep bite, sustained by a significantly high amplitude of EMG activity in masticatory muscles together with high repetitivity and low variability of the chewing pattern (Throckmorton *et al.*, 2001; Piancino *et al.,* 2013).

Equilibrium between repetitivity and variability constitutes an alternation of opposites, a typical feature of rhythmic movements that underpins all vital functions. This is, therefore, the intrinsic feature of normal healthy mastication and is also the reason for the difficulties encountered when attempting to use the mathematical–statistical calculations normally adopted in bioengineering. Analytical study of masticatory function requires a specific bioengineering approach to calculate the average chewing cycle, and the adoption of complex mathematical–statistical laws to correctly evaluate numeric, kinetic, and EMG data. The technical and statistical will not be described in this book being published in the scientific literature; this book is intended for practical clinical understanding of masticatory function. The characteristics of a chewing pattern that are described in the following pages refer to the study of the particular malocclusion to which this book is dedicated: the unilateral posterior and anterior crossbite. Thus, this book is not intended as a guide to mastication in all malocclusions, but is specifically dedicated to explaining the effects of unilateral posterior crossbite, outlining some logical and coherent concepts. The study of unilateral posterior crossbite is useful for evaluating the direct occlusal influence on chewing patterns and neuromuscular activity.

2.5.3 Diagnostic indices of chewing patterns

So far, we have described the characteristics of masticatory function, focusing on the tables of overlapping chewing cycles one by one. This aspect is important in order to understand the concepts of symmetry and specularity, variability and repetitivity, and the physiological pattern. However, in light of the complexity of this subject and its constant evolution, the aid of computer technology is essential in analyzing chewing patterns. From the outset, research studies set out to identify numeric indices with clinical significance and, to this end, bespoke software was created that automatically analyzed homogeneous mastication samples to provide average values of selected numeric indices from a sizeable number of chewing cycles.

The significance of these numeric indices will be explained in this chapter. They have been subdivided into the following types:

- vectorial;
- dimensional;
- positional.

From this point on, they will be illustrated by tracking of individual overlapping cycles, joined by tracking of averages, supplied by computer means.

2.5.3.1 *Vectorial indices*
2.5.3.1.1 *Closing direction* (Figure 2.15)

- *Definition.*
  The direction of closure is represented by the vector of the closing pattern in the last phase of the chewing cycle. It may be clockwise or anti-clockwise, according to the bolus side.

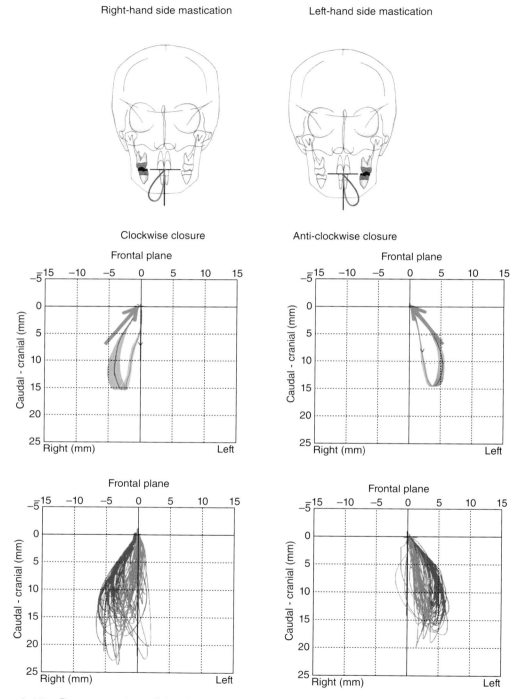

Figure 2.15 Representation of the direction of the tracing of closure: clockwise during chewing on the right side; anti-clockwise during chewing on the left side. Green tracings: opening; red tracings: closing.

- *Physiological characteristics.*
  The importance of closing direction, was first understood and masterfully described by A. Lewin

  The most important part of the chewing pattern, from an efficiency point of view, is undoubtedly the closing shift, in particular during the second phase of closure when approaching functional occlusion.

  The physiological pattern on the frontal plane is characterized by a mandibular shift downwards during the opening phase, by a lateral mandibular glide toward the bolus side during the first phase of closure, and by a medial shift during the second phase of closure and transcuspidal and intercuspidal phases. One very important physiological parameter for the evaluation of chewing patterns is the closure direction. When analyzing the chewing pattern from in front of the patient (and not from behind), *during mastication on the right-hand side, chewing cycles display a clockwise closure direction.* Generally, the axis is inclined to the right, and most chewing cycles develop on the bolus side on the right.

  Conversely, *during mastication on the left-hand side, chewing cycles display an anti-clockwise closure direction.* Generally, the axis is inclined to the left, and most chewing cycles develop on the bolus side on the left. *The direction of the last stage of closure is an important indicator of chewing pattern characteristics and balanced mastication.*

  The physiological direction of closure displays the symmetry and specularity of masticatory movement which permits symmetric effort and harmony of the stomatognathic system parts. When the closure direction changes and inverts on one side only, the mirrored quality is lost, as is the symmetrical movement. In fact, when the closure direction is reverse (i.e. it becomes anti-clockwise with the right-hand bolus), the chewing pattern becomes totally abnormal – with near-clashes of opening and closing phases, development along the vertical axis area, and possible cross-over of opening and closing paths (possibly on multiple occasions).

  The closing direction is a true indicator of changes to chewing cycles – there is no cycle with reverse closing direction and physiological patterns, not at any age or in any condition. A high percentage of reverse-sequence chewing cycles calls for diagnosis and treatment. The reverse closure direction is a vital clinical indicator. Unfortunately, some articles in the literature are biased and based on errors, which has led to much confusion on this issue. We will look further at this in Chapter 4. For the moment, we underline that *the mirrored property of the closing direction is an indicator of healthy symmetric chewing function.*

2.5.3.1.2 *Closing angle* (Figure 2.16)

In normal healthy occlusion and physiological stomatognathic activity, the mandible opens along the vertical axis and glides laterally from the bolus side to the point of maximum opening; in the closure phase it returns upward until maximum functional intercuspation is reached (Figure 2.17).

The closing angle is one of the most important vector indicators of a chewing cycle from a clinical point of view. It represents the inclination with which the mandibular and vestibular cuspids of the lower molars and premolars approach the bolus and/or the occlusal surface of teeth on the opposing upper arch, before entering the transcuspid and intercuspid stages of mastication dedicated to the grinding of the bolus. Its *specularity and symmetry* during mastication on the right-hand side compared with the left-hand side are, once again, *important clinical signs of functional balance.*

- *Definition.*
  The closing angle is identified by the tangent line in the last part of the closing pattern compared with the horizontal or vertical axis.

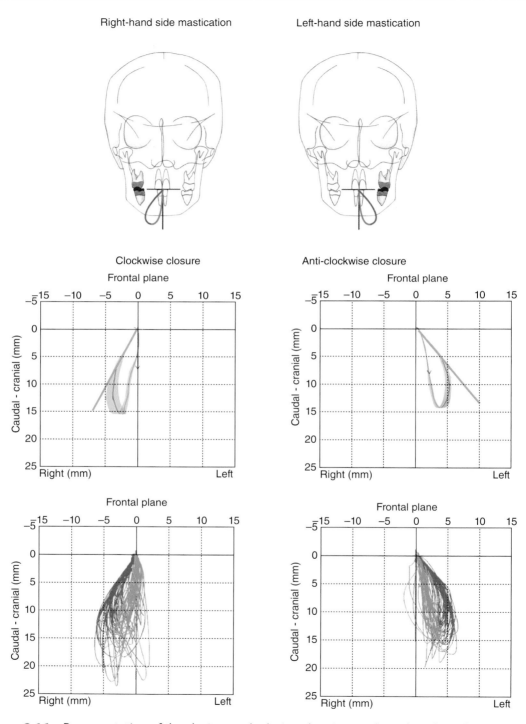

Figure 2.16 Representation of the closing angle during chewing on the right side and on the left side. Green tracings: opening; red tracings: closing.

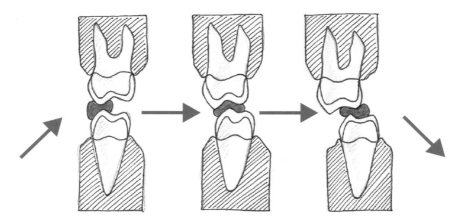

Figure 2.17 In physiological conditions, the mandible deviates laterally, toward the bolus side, and then, during closure, medially through the transcuspal and intercuspal phases of mastication. *Source:* Redrawn from A. Lewin (1985) with the permission of Quintessence Publishing.

- *Pathophysiology characteristics.*

  In normal physiological conditions, the closing angle displays a variable inclination compared with the vertical axis. This value is lower during mastication of a soft bolus than of a hard bolus (in the same patient). The closing angle is identified in the second phase of closure, the bolus-grinding stage, which has also been defined as the "power phase of closure" (Morquette et al., 2012). Together with the closing direction (described earlier), this is an important clinical indicator as it reveals the angle with which the mandible reaches maximum intercuspation.

  This has been described by A. Lewin as one of the parameters of masticatory efficiency (Wilding and Lewin, 1991a,b, 1994; Wilding et al., 1992). The further the closing angle remains from the vertical axis (i.e. the greater the angle with which the mandible reaches the bolus), the more efficient will the masticatory function be. The nearer the closing angle remains to the vertical axis (i.e. the greater the proximity of the mandible to the bolus and the upper cuspids near or along the vertical axis), the less efficient will mastication be. To support this point, we know that the amplitude of the closing angle changes according to the type of bolus. During mastication of a hard bolus, which requires extra masticatory effort, the closing angle moves away from the vertical axis and the mandible reaches the bolus with a greater angle trajectory than the vertical axis (with the size of the angle depending on how much effort is required for mastication). On the contrary, during mastication of a soft bolus, the closing angle is nearer the vertical axis but still (in normal conditions) on the bolus side.

  As mastication is a rhythmic functional movement, variability and unique features will manifest in each individual. For a reliable clinical analysis of chewing patterns (avoiding bias caused by variability) we should *evaluate the electrognathography and EMG data using a methodology that is not absolute and independent in itself but relative and connected to other contexts.* Thus, by comparing the values collected during mastication of a soft bolus with those of a hard bolus, we can determine whether the patient's stomatognathic system is in proper working order or whether there are some problems connected to adjustment. By repeating the test at a later moment in time (or after treatment), we can again compare the new results with the previous values to determine whether some improvement or deterioration has taken place.

Apart from the variations in mastication of different bolus types, specularity and symmetry of the closing angle/direction during mastication are significant clinical indicators and important for functional equilibrium, particularly throughout the childhood years of growth and development, but also in adulthood. In fact, the muscular effort required by efficient mastication represents the functional matrix described by Moss (i.e. the force that drives the development of a child's cranial structure). If muscular effort is asymmetrically distributed, the growth and development will be discordant, worsening over time and irreversible once the period of growth has stopped (Moss, 1968). In adulthood, discordance no longer has an effect on growth but it does impact the functional compensation caused by asymmetry that leads to wear and tear and hyperactivity of some structures, which may heighten the risk of algic diseases.

This should be the approach if we want to assign clinical significance to masticatory function. Considering solely the direction and angle of closure on one side has little sense; we must, instead, perform a bilateral comparative evaluation of these parameters that reveal unequivocally the symmetry or asymmetry of a pattern, and the neuromuscular effort involved. Let us not forget that mastication, in normal physiological conditions, is a rhythmic, alternating, and harmonious movement occurring many times every day. There are many events or conditions that may disrupt its balance, causing asymmetric chewing action, and these need to be diagnosed in order to understand the etiopathogenesis of the dysfunction and/or malocclusion.

We will see in Chapter 4 that abnormal cycles known as "reverse sequence" (due to their inverse closing direction) are marked by a severely altered closing angle (almost vertical) opposite the bolus side, and we will see also how the restoration and realignment of symmetry in the closing angle (following the correction of the closing direction of the chewing cycle) is essential in re-establishing physiologically balanced masticatory function.

The physiological orthodontic movement of teeth consistent with bone and muscles is the way to "cure" the patient's stomatognathic system – finally progressing to a true "medical treatment" of the masticatory function.

2.5.3.2 Dimensional indices: height and width (Figure 2.18)

In normal physiological conditions of occlusion and stomatognathic functioning, the height and width of the chewing pattern are *referential indicators of the morphological character of the pattern, its efficiency, and its capacity to adjust to different bolus types*. As explained for the direction and angle of closure, specularity and symmetry of height and width are again significant clinical indicators of functional equilibrium.

- *Definitions.*
  Height: distance between the point of functional intercuspation and the point where the opening turns to closure.
  Width: distance between the opening and closing tracks at the point of maximum width of the chewing cycle, perpendicular to the axis of the chewing cycle.
- *Physiological characteristics.*
  As previously stated for the closing angle, for height and width, too, electrognathographic data must always be read in a relative (not absolute) sense. Thus, it is the *comparison between values achieved during mastication of a soft bolus with that of a hard bolus* that will enable us to understand whether the patient's stomatognathic system is functionally balanced or whether it has problems connected to adjustment. Repetition of the exam at a later date or

Mastication on the right-hand side   Mastication on the left-hand side

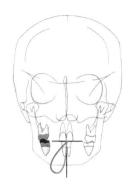   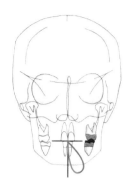

Clockwise closure   Anti-clockwise closing direction

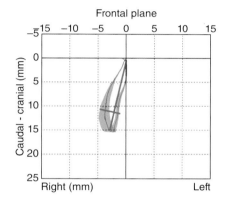   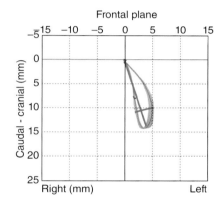

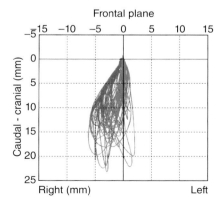   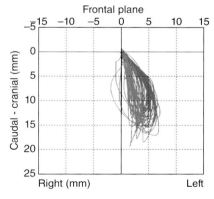

Figure 2.18   Representation of the height and width of the chewing pattern during chewing on the right side and on the left side. Green tracings: opening; red tracings: closing.

after therapy will allow a comparison with the preceding results to diagnose the improvement or worsening of the indices.

In fact, while a soft bolus is being chewed, both the height and width of the chewing cycle are inferior to those during mastication of a hard bolus. Just as with the closing angle, the "maximum height and width" parameters change and adapt to the characteristics of the bolus and, thus, of the efficiency requirements of mastication.

The height and width are also indices of adjustment to load and masticatory efficiency (Lewin, 1985). They indicate the health status of the structures and the good coordination of the stomatognathic system. Motor programming of the masticatory pattern with *a hard bolus* (which involves a *greater height and width of the cycle* to achieve improved efficiency and greater force in grinding the bolus) can occur only if the stomatognathic structures (occlusion, muscles, TMJ movement) are biologically healthy (devoid of harmful input from occlusion, pain, or muscle fatigue) and physiologically coordinated (correct dental guide, symmetrical occlusion, symmetrical muscular activity, homogeneous and symmetric glide movement of the joint).

Conversely, a tight chewing cycle – repetitive, limited in height and width – indicates a stomatognathic system with severely limited movement. Furthermore, *the failure of the chewing cycle to increase in height and width during mastication of hard bolus as opposed to a soft bolus indicates a limited ability to adjust to load*; in other words, of a stomatognathic apparatus that is "imprisoned" and immobilized in a pattern unable to change or adapt. In such cases, one of the most important features of mastication, its variability and ability to adapt, is lost and there is the risk of jaw bone, TMJ, and muscular overloading.

One more important point in order to understand the clinical usefulness of the study of mastication: as we will see later, some parameters are directly linked to dental malocclusion and the diagnosis is straightforward, whilst others (such as a limited ability to adjust to load) can be viewed as *early signs of functional difficulty* that may not yet be available to clinical diagnosis or other instrumental analysis.

2.5.3.3 *Positional index: lateral shift* (Figure 2.19)

The lateral shift is a positional index of the chewing cycle; that is, an indicator that reveals the capacity for lateral shifting of the mandible on the frontal plane. Regardless of the width or height of the masticatory cycle, the shift can occur along the vertical axis or more laterally toward the bolus side. In the event of a pathological condition, it can occur on the contralateral side. The width of the pattern is an intrinsic parameter of the masticatory cycle, but it is also necessary to evaluate its spatial position in order to diagnose the capacity of mandibular shift, which reveals the state of muscular and joint functioning.

- *Definition.*
  The lateral shift is the most distant point from the track of closure of the vertical axis.
     In normal physiological conditions, the distance of the closing path of mastication from the vertical axis matches the width of the chewing cycle.
- *Clinical interpretation.*
  The lateral shift *defines the capacity of the mandible to move on the bolus side*. In normal physiological conditions the mandible moves from the bolus side both during mastication directed exclusively either right or left and during free mastication directed alternately to both right and left. In normal conditions, the mandible shifts laterally in direction proportional to the width of the cycle (which we have already identified as an efficiency parameter). However, in abnormal conditions, there may be a very tight pattern with a fixed level of lateral shift. In such cases, the opening path overlaps and/or is very close to the closing track. The direction

of closure might be physiological and the efficiency of the chewing cycle maintained, but the patient's occlusal/muscular/articular characteristics must be evaluated and analyzed further with clinical tests and tools.

The most important clinical observation to be made regarding lateral shift is always the search for specularity and symmetry of the movement. In physiological conditions, the lateral shift of the mandible is symmetric.

Cases may occur where the chewing pattern displays normal morphology but the mandible shifts on one side only. In such cases, the "lateral shift" positional index will reveal evident asymmetry between the sides, indicating that the mandible is functionally unable to move from one side. This positional asymmetry in the chewing pattern often appears in the presence of crossbite due to the altered chewing cycle, as we will see later, but it may also appear in other occlusal and articular conditions, and may be an early warning sign of imbalanced masticatory function requiring careful clinical diagnosis. Asymmetry of the chewing pattern must always be seriously evaluated because it may be a condition that continues to worsen over time and, as mastication is a daily action, this may damage the system and allow the arrival of algic or dysfunctional pathologies.

2.5.3.4 Parameters of efficiency of the chewing pattern

Establishing the efficiency of the masticatory cycle according to electrognathographic tracking is no easy matter, but by learning to relate the different aspects of the pattern whilst avoiding univocal and sectorial claims it becomes possible to diagnose efficiency levels.

One of the last scientific articles published by A. Lewin was dedicated to the study of parameters that indicate efficiency levels of mastication, and today this still provides a point of reference for those studying masticatory function (Wilding and Lewin, 1994). *Lewin identified four parameters of masticatory efficiency and underlined the fact that any one single parameter is not enough to establish said levels.*

The four parameters identified are:

1. the angle of closure
2. the area
3. the height
4. the width.

To evaluate the validity of prosthetic rehabilitation, many studies rely on analysis of the shredding of sifted bolus (Optosil®). Along similar lines, Lepley *et al.* (2010) published an article relating the parameters of efficiency of the masticatory cycle with an analysis of bolus shredding (a protocol used for the study of mastication in patients with prosthetic implants), confirming that a more thoroughly shredded bolus will lead to higher efficiency values in the masticatory cycle. Of course, the analysis of parameters of chewing patterns is a more precise and complete indicator than the shredding of Optosil.

If the study of mastication is to have a diagnostic and therapeutic clinical significance, we must not make the mistake of considering masticatory function exclusively from the point of view of efficiency. *Efficiency is certainly an important parameter, but the issues of symmetry and neuromuscular equilibrium are of vital importance, for preserving a healthy stomatognathic system.* This is because there is significant muscular effort during mastication, which can influence structural and cognitive growth in the period of development (Kawahata *et al.*, 2014). *The effects of functional compensation to an asymmetrical structural pathology recur throughout the entire stomatognathic system over time, even though in the initial phase masticatory efficiency may seem to be maintained.*

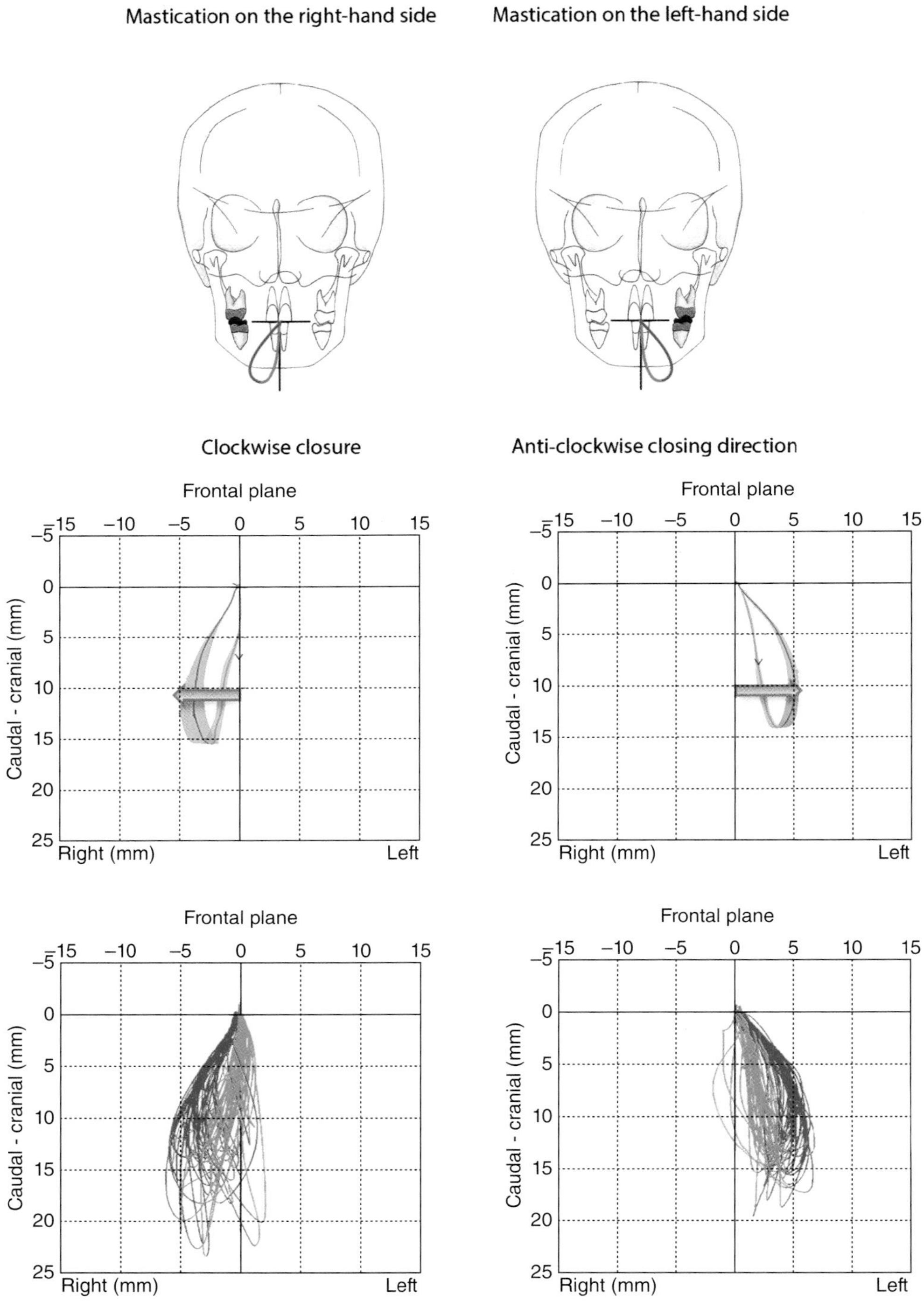

Figure 2.19 Representation of the lateral shift of the chewing pattern during chewing on the right side and on the left side. Green tracings: opening; red tracings: closing.

Masticatory efficiency is an important parameter, but alone it is not enough: symmetry and coordination between the two sides are fundamental for the future health of the stomatognathic structures.

2.5.2.4.1 Mastication in the premolar and molar areas

As described by R. Slavicek, occlusion can be divided into different areas on the basis of their allocated functions. The front area, defined by Slavicek as a real sensory organ, is characterized by highly concentrated and specialized periodontal receptors. It is responsible for static and dynamic postural control of the mandible throughout space. The role of front and canine teeth in mastication is that of controlling mandibular position in space. On the contrary, the role of the posterior occlusal area in mastication is active and direct; that is, the teeth of the back area are dedicated to mastication and the grinding of food. The posterior occlusal region, in its strictest sense, comprises the first, second, and third molars, with the first and second premolars acting as an area of transition between the front and back areas (Slavicek, 2002).

This anatomical subdivision has functional foundations that have been described by A. Lewin in his studies on mastication. Chewing cycles that occur during mastication in the premolar region are visibly more narrow than those of the molar region, whether with a hard or soft bolus. In other words, when chewing in the premolar region, the area between the opening and closing tracks is smaller, the closing angle is more vertical and the cycle height is inferior to that of the chewing cycle during mastication in the molar area. All the parameters mentioned, present simultaneously, are indices of reduced masticatory efficiency (Wilding and Lewin, 1991a, b, 1992, 1994; Hashii *et al.*, 2009). This means that mastication in the premolar area is less efficient, while in the molar area it is much more efficient and this is in agreement with the functional role of the regions of the occlusion.

2.5.3.5 Mastication of soft and hard bolus: adjustment to load (Figure 2.20)

The chewing pattern's ability to adjust to the type of bolus is evidence of the precise neural control of the masticatory pattern and is a vital clinical indicator of healthy functioning of the stomatognathic system.

The masticatory pattern that evolves during chewing of a soft bolus is clearly different from that developed during chewing of a hard bolus. The most suitable type of pattern is selected according to peripheral input, beginning with the receptors of the stomatognathic system, which, as we will see, are highly concentrated, sensitive and specialized, and in direct contact with the nuclei of the central nervous system. Thanks to these characteristics, highly precise data are conveyed to the cortex on the type of bolus, its dimensions, and its taste consistency. According to this data, the most suitable chewing pattern will be adopted in order to grind the bolus with maximum efficiency and minimum energy consumption. In physiological conditions, the pattern developed during mastication of a soft bolus is tighter, of a lower height/smaller area, and with a more vertical trajectory of the occlusal phase of the closing pattern than during mastication of a hard bolus. All the parameters of efficiency show that the chewing pattern of the soft bolus is less efficient compared with the chewing pattern of the hard bolus, which demonstrates greater height, width, and closure angle. As previously explained, the ability to adjust to load is an important clinical data.

The apex of the chewing cycle of a soft bolus (near maximum intercuspation) is a type of point source as the soft bolus presents minimal resistance and allows the cuspids to approach maximum intercuspation. On the other hand, a hard bolus offers significant resistance and keeps the mandible far from maximum intercuspation, undergoing a more evident transcuspal phase. Gradually, as the hard bolus is worn down, the cycle tends to become tighter and shorter, approaching by degrees the point of maximum intercuspation. The standard exam of masticatory cycles involves recording results with both a soft and hard bolus, from which a comparative analysis of the two patterns will reveal the patient's capacity to adjust to load (Piancino *et al.*, 2005, 2006, 2007, 2008).

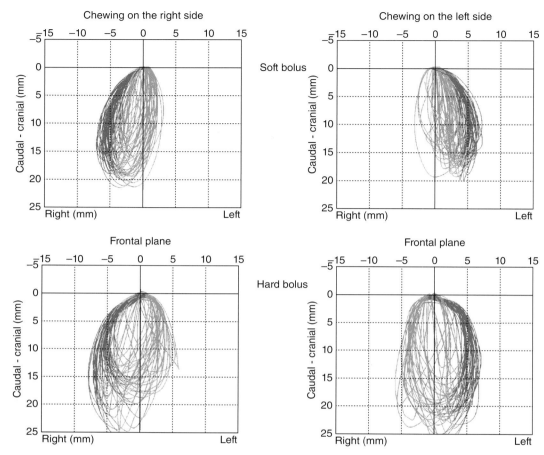

Figure 2.20 Overlapping chewing patterns during chewing a soft bolus (*top*) and hard bolus (*bottom*) on the right and left side. Green tracings: opening; red tracings: closing.

References

Bracco P, Anastasi G, Piancino MG, *et al.* (2010) Hemispheric prevalence during chewing in normal right-handed and left-handed subjects: a functional magnetic resonance imaging preliminary study. *Cranio* 28(2), 114–121.

Ferrario V, Piancino MG, Dellavia C, *et al.* (2006) Quantitative analysis of the variability of unilateral chewing movements in young adults. *Cranio* 24(4), 274–282.

Gibbs CH, Lundeen HC, Mahan PE, Fujimoto J. (1981a) Chewing movements in relation to border movements at the first molar. *J Prosthet Dent* 46(3), 308–322.

Gibbs CH, Mahan PE, Lundeen HC, *et al.* (1981b) Occlusal forces during chewing and swallowing as measured by sound transmission. *J Prosthet Dent* 46(4), 443–449.

Gibbs CH, Mahan PE, Lundeen HC, *et al.* (1981c) Occlusal forces during chewing – influences of biting strength and food consistency. *J Prosthet Dent* 46(5), 561–567.

Gibbs CH, Wickwire NA, Jacobson AP, *et al.* (1982) Comparison of typical chewing patterns in normal children and adults. *J Am Dent Assoc* 105(1), 33–42.

Hashii K, Tomida M, Yamashita S. (2009) Influence of changing the chewing region on mandibular movement. *Aust Dent J* 54(1), 38–44.

Hirano Y, Obata T, Kashikura K, *et al*. (2008) Effects of chewing in working memory processing. *Neurosci Lett* 436(2), 189–192.

Ingervall B, Carlsson GE, Thilander B (1976) Postnatal development of the human temporomandibular joint. II. A microradiographic study. *Acta Odontol Scand* 34(3), 133–139.

Kandel ER, Schwartz JH, Jessel TM, *et al*. (eds) (2012) *Principles of neural science*, 5th edn. McGraw-Hill, New York.

Katsavrias E, Dibbets JMH. (2001) The growth of articular eminence height during craniofacial growth period. *Cranio* 19, 13–20.

Kawahata M, Ono Y, Ohno A, *et al*. (2014) Loss of molars early in life develops behavioral lateralization and impairs hippocampus-dependent recognition memory. *BMC Neurosci* 15, 4.

Lepley C, Throckmorton G, Parker S, Buschang PH. (2010) Masticatory performance and chewing cycle kinematics – are they related? *Angle Orthod* 80(2), 295–301.

Lewin A. (1985) *Electrognathographics. An atlas for diagnostic procedures and interpretation*. Quintessence, Berlin.

Lewin A, Evans WG, Booth JL, Howes DG. (1995) Constrained and unconstrained postures of the mandible – a break with tradition? *Ann Acad Med Singapore* 24(1), 3–10.

Lundeen HC, Gibbs CH. (1982) *Advances in occlusion*. J. Wright–PSG, Boston, MA.

Morquette P, Lavoie R, Fhima MD, *et al*. (2012) Generation of the masticatory central pattern and its modulation by sensory feedback. *Prog Neurobiol* 96(3), 340–355.

Moss ML. (1968) A theoretical analysis of the functional matrix. *Acta Biotheor* 18(1), 195–202.

Naeije M, Hofman N. (2003) Biomechanics of the human temporomandibular joint during chewing. *J Dent Res* 82(7), 528–531.

Neff P. (1999) *TMJ occlusion and function*. Georgetown University School of Dentistry, Washington, DC. http://peterneffdds.com/blog, http://www.amazon.com/TMJ-occlusion-function-Peter-Neff/dp/B0006RE5SK (accessed October 2, 2015).

Nerder PH, Bakke M, Solow B. (1999) The functional shift of the mandible in unilateral posterior crossbite and the adaptation of the temporomandibular joints: a pilot study. *Eur J Orthod* 21(2), 155–166.

Nitzan DW. (2002) Temporomandibular joint "open lock" versus condylar dislocation: signs and symptoms, imaging, treatment, and pathogenesis. *J Oral Maxillofac Surg* 60(5), 506–511.

Nitzan DW. (2003) "Friction and adhesive forces" – possible underlying causes for temporomandibular joint internal derangement. *Cells Tissues Organs* 174(1–2), 6–16.

Nitzan DW, Etsion I. (2002) Adhesive force: the underlying cause of the disc anchorage to the fossa and/or eminence in the temporomandibular joint-a new concept. *Int J Oral Maxillofac Surg* 31(1), 94–99.

Nitzan DW, Kreiner B, Zeltser R. (2004) TMJ lubrication system: its effect on the joint function, dysfunction, and treatment approach. *Compend Contin Educ Dent* 25(6), 437–438, 440, 443–444 passim; quiz 449, 471.

Piancino MG, Talpone F, Bole T, *et al*. (2005) Electromyographic evaluation of neuromuscular co-ordination during chewing in a subject with organic occlusion. *Min Stomatol* 54(6), 379–387.

Piancino MG, Talpone F, Dalmasso P, *et al*. (2006) Reverse-sequencing chewing patterns before and after treatment of children with a unilateral posterior crossbite. *Eur J Orthod* 28(5), 480–484.

Piancino MG, Farina D, Merlo A, *et al*. (2007) Early treatment with "function generating bite" of a left unilateral posterior cross-bite: chewing pattern before and after therapy with FGB. *Int J Orthod Milwaukee* 18(2), 33–38.

Piancino MG, Bracco P, Vallelonga T, *et al*. (2008) Effect of bolus hardness on the chewing pattern and activation of masticatory muscles in subjects with normal dental occlusion. *J Electromyogr Kinesiol* 18(6), 931–937.

Piancino MG, Farina D, Talpone F, *et al*. (2009) Muscular activation during reverse and non-reverse chewing cycles in unilateral posterior crossbite. *Eur J Oral Sci* 117(2), 122–128.

Piancino MG, Vallelonga T, Debernardi C, Bracco P. (2013) Deep bite: a case report with chewing pattern and electromyographic activity before and after therapy with function generating bite. *Eur J Paediatr Dent* 14(2), 156–159.

Pinto AS, Buschang PH, Throckmorton GS, Chen P. (2001) Morphological and positional asymmetries of young children with functional unilateral posterior crossbite. *Am J Orthod Dentofacial Orthop* 120(5), 513–520.

Purves D, Augustine GJ, Fitzpatrick, *et al.* (2000) *Neuroscienze* (trans. RLucchi, APoli, MVirgili). Zanichelli, Bologna.

Ronnerman A, Thilander B. (1978) Facial and dental arch morphology in children with and without early loss of deciduous molars. *Am J Orthod* 73(1), 47–58.

Slavicek R. (2002) *The masticatory organ: functions and dysfunctions.* Gamma Medizinisch-wissenschaftliche Fortbildung-AG, Klosterneuburg.

Takada T, Miyamoto T. (2004) A fronto-parietal network for chewing of gum: a study on human subjects with functional magnetic resonance imaging. *Neurosci Lett* 360(3), 137–140.

Thilander B. (2000) Orthodontic relapse versus natural development. *Am J Orthod Dentofacial Orthop* 117(5), 562–563.

Thilander B, Lennartsson B. (2002) A study of children with unilateral posterior crossbite, treated and untreated, in the deciduous dentition – occlusal and skeletal characteristics of significance in predicting the long-term outcome. *J Orofac Orthop* 63(5), 371–383.

Thilander B, Carlsson GE, Ingerval B. (1976) Postnatal development of the human temporomandibular joint. I. A histological study. *Acta Odont Scand* 34, 117–126.

Thilander B, Rubio G, Pena L, de Mayorga C. (2002) Prevalence of temporomandibular dysfunction and its association with malocclusion in children and adolescents: an epidemiologic study related to specified stages of dental development. *Angle Orthod* 72(2), 146–154.

Throckmorton GS, Buschang PH, Hayasaki H, Santos Pinto A (2001) Changes in the masticatory cycle following treatment of posterior unilateral crossbite in children. *Am J Orthod Dentofacial Orthop* 120, 521–529.

Wilding RJ, Lewin A. (1991a) A computer analysis of normal human masticatory movements recorded with a Sirognathograph. *Arch Oral Biol* 36(1), 65–75.

Wilding RJ, Lewin A (1991b) A model for optimum functional human jaw movements based on values associated with preferred chewing patterns. *Arch Oral Biol* 36(7), 519–523.

Wilding RJ, Lewin A. (1994) The determination of optimal human jaw movements based on their association with chewing performance. *Arch Oral Biol* 39(4), 333–343.

Wilding RJ, Adams LP, Lewin A. (1992) Absence of association between a preferred chewing side and its area of functional occlusal contact in the human dentition. *Arch Oral Biol* 37(5), 423–428.

Chapter 3

Physiology of Mastication: Neuromuscular Control of Masticatory Function

Contents

Understanding Masticatory Function in Unilateral Crossbites, First Edition. Maria Grazia Piancino and Stephanos Kyrkanides.
© 2016 John Wiley & Sons, Inc. Published 2016 by John Wiley & Sons, Inc.

3.1 Importance of the motor activity (Figure 3.1)

As mentioned in the introduction to Chapters 1 and 2, understanding of the neuromuscular control of mastication is important in order to comprehend this function. In fact, *teeth are the dominant structure in the stomatognathic system and, via this rigid structure and their sensorial/proprioceptive input, all functional processes of the masticatory system are determined.* All programs for analyzing chewing patterns are established on the basis of this understanding. However, a *comprehension of neuromuscular control of mastication* is fundamental not only from a research point of view regarding mastication itself, but also, and above all, from a clinical point of view *to understand the compensatory measures and adjustments that the system makes in order to protect biological structures.*

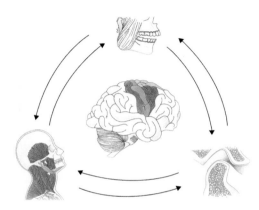

The system is able *to adapt its function and compensate faults* (i.e., malocclusions, traumas, growth alterations), but *it is not able to correct the fault.* Comprehension of adjustments and/or dynamic compensatory measures, which result from structural faults and which in turn condition growth, is the first step toward *understanding and diagnosing the etiopathogenesis of functional malocclusions, and choosing the appropriate treatment in full respect of tissues biology and physiological condition of the stomatognathic system* (Moss, 1968; Enlow, 1986). This approach to the pathology of occlusion is medical, as it logically should be, particularly when dealing with cranial growth in developmental age. However, such a beneficial approach is still unfortunately the prerogative of too few people, as the conviction reigns that this issue is simply too complex. In reality, this is the approach that allows a coherent understanding of the etiopathogenesis of associated occlusal and neuromuscular alterations. We hope that this book may be of assistance to students and professionals in the fields of dentistry, and other related areas, in helping them to understand neuromuscular control of mastication and its influence on the harmonious growth of the cranial skeletal structure, and both in adulthood and old age.

Before describing the general characteristics of the neuromuscular system, in order to give a widespread overview of the topic without sectorializing, we believe it necessary to dedicate a few lines to *recent neurological evolution that has opened up new horizons and overcome the static subdivisions of the nervous system*, allowing an understanding of multidisciplinary effects of neuromuscular control of the stomatognathic system.

In the 1980s, research in the field of neuroscience was subdivided into separate areas of perception (peripheral

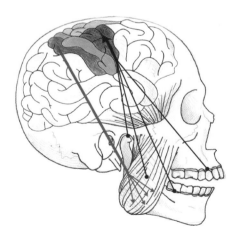

Figure 3.1 Motor control of masticatory function. The stomatognathic system: relationships between dental occlusion, TMJ, and neuromuscular control. *Source for the muscles:* Redrawn from Neff (1999). *Source for the brain:* Redrawn from Purves *et al.* (2000). Reproduced with permission of Sinauer Associates.

input, sensorial system), action (muscular activation, motor system), and cognitive activity (planning, thought). Actually, we know that our world experience is unitary and, for the brain, perception and action constitute a single unit. A first step in this sense occurred when the *concept of motor homunculus*, which statically associated cerebral areas with precise anatomic structures, *was overcome*. The motor cortex seems to be organized in *columns formed by cell groups capable of controlling a simple movement, which may involve different muscles as well*. The result is a driving unit that can be controlled by different columns in an apparently confused complex of cortical areas. In other words, motor cortex organization is not static but is based on functional and dynamic features.

Of notable significance and of interest in the dental field also, is the *recent discovery of mirror neurons* by a workgroup led by G. Rizzolati of the University of Parma (Italy). Mirror neurons were originally discovered in the ventral premotor cortex of the macaw, a species that is distinctly social, like humans. These motor neurons are able *to transform the action from a (visual) sensorial form to a motor form*. The same neurons that are activated during the action of a subject are activated also in the observer, without the observer completing any type of action. The observer, thanks to the activation of this chain, acquires a motor representation of the entire action that the agent intends to carry out. In this way, the intention can be understood, to predict the agent's future behavior. This shows how sensory, motor, and cognitive systems are closely linked. Mirror neurons displayed signs of their presence many years before being discovered (Iacoboni, 2008), but to understand their features it was necessary to eliminate the barrier that kept the sensory, motor, and cognitive systems separate from each other. Many experiments showed how a mirror mechanism is present in humans in the inferior parietal lobule, in the ventral premotor area, and the posterior area of the inferior frontal gyrus (Gallese *et al.*, 1996; Rizzolatti *et al.*, 1996; Rizzolatti and Craighero, 2004; Fogassi *et al.*, 2005; Rizzolatti and Sinigaglia, 2010).

Human data (as for monkeys) show that the *intention underlying the action performed by others is perceived and understood thanks to the mirror system*. Obviously, this does not mean that the mirror mechanism is the only one that allows us to understand the intention of others; there are other mechanisms that achieve the same goal, such as inferential reasoning. However, the mirror system offers a different, experiential knowledge based on the circuit activity that we adopt when we ourselves perform the action. The generally accepted hypothesis is that *mirror neurons are necessary for immediate comprehension of other actions. The motor act evokes the necessary motor program in the observer in order to perform it, and this allows the cognitive comprehension of everything around us.* In other words, the sensorial, motor and cognitive systems constantly interact with each other.

At this point, the following question is justified: when the observer looks at an action that they know, is the mirror system facilitated? Research would seem to confirm so, showing that the mirror system encodes the motor acts performed by others on the basis of the observer's store of motor experience; the more this is developed, the more efficient the system becomes. And, so, *it is motor learning (as opposed to visual experience) that is the main factor responsible for activating the mirror system* (Rizzolatti and Craighero, 2004; Rizzolatti and Sinigaglia, 2010); the intention underlying the action performed by others is comprehended thanks to the mirror system and to the motor experience of the subject. *The motor experience is important for cognitive activity*.

It seems logical, then, that the mirror system be involved in more advanced human processes. In fact, studies have been carried out into the involvement of the mirror system in language and learning by imitation, which is a cornerstone of childhood physiological development. There are convincing experimental tests, based on studies of functional resonance, which suggest the mirror system is involved both in the immediate repetition of actions performed by others and in the learning of new motor patterns. There is, however, an important difference between the two cases. Immediate repetition of an act performed by others activates the mirror system without involving higher order cortical areas. However, learning by imitation (typical and fundamental for human development) occurs via a more complex mechanism, which involves not only the mirror system but also the prefrontal lobe (Rizzolatti *et al.*, 1996, Rizzolatti and Craighero, 2004, Rizzolatti and Sinigaglia, 2010).

The activity of mirror neurons is fundamental in recognizing the intentions and emotions of others, for imitative learning in the age of growth, and for verbal communication and language; it underpins social and emotional relationships, and it is based on motor experience.

The section of this book dedicated to the revolutionary discovery of mirror neurons is not coincidental but it is due to the fact that, in light of the new discoveries and a new neurological approach, the hypothesis seems likely that a motor act like mastication (which involves muscles in an important role from the point of view of coordination, EMG amplitude, contraction force, rhythm, and daily repetitivity) may exert *a direct influence (particularly during growth) not only on the harmonious growth of the cranium*, but also on the harmonious cognitive development of the child, conditioning the equilibrium and future function of the stomatognathic system together with the cognitive capacities. The fact that mastication involves cephalic muscles in a coordinated manner, and that its equilibrium in the age of development may underpin not only harmonious skeletal and joint growth but also advanced development of cognitive skills, is finally emerging as the focus of general and clinical research studies.

In fact, recent articles demonstrate that early extraction and asymmetry of a molar tooth in growing animals (mouse) determines not only an alteration to masticatory function but to cognitive function as well, particularly regarding attention span and memory, involving the prefrontal cortex and hippocampus (Kawahata *et al.*, 2014; Teixeira *et al.*, 2014). Moreover, a recent revision of the literature regarding the effects of masticatory changes on cognitive function in laboratory animals and humans concluded that the epidemiological data suggest *a positive correlation between alterations to mastication and the mechanisms underlying some cognitive skills* (Smith, 2010; Davidson, 2011; Onyper *et al.*, 2011; Hirano *et al.*, 2013; Yu *et al.*, 2013). Also, many articles have been dedicated to proving the clear positive *influence of mastication in humans*, whether with prosthetics or natural dentition, *on cognitive activity in patients in old age* (Narita *et al.*, 2009; Kawanishi *et al.*, 2010; Ono *et al.*, 2010; Lexomboon *et al.*, 2012; Hansson *et al.*, 2013; Kimura *et al.*, 2013; Shoi *et al.*, 2014).

However, there is also evidence in *the developmental age*. In fact, *a study evaluating a group of young patients between 15 and 25 years of age with posterior crossbite*, compared with a control group without malocclusions, showed a significant association between the malocclusion, the functional alterations, and the cognitive assessment (Johnston *et al.*, 2012; Masood *et al.*, 2014; Kawahata *et al.*, 2014).

It seems increasingly clear, therefore, that there is *a relationship between sensory-motor and cognitive forms of activity* (Figure 3.1). From this point of view, a healthy stomatognathic system is important because it is the actor of the masticatory function and it infers the absence of incongruous peripheral stimuli that fire imbalanced muscular activity and self-regenerating loops that worsen continually; it means a better control of stress impacting the stomatognathic system, greater emotional stability, and improved cognitive skills (Masood *et al.*, 2014). This does not mean that the stomatognathic system is at the crossroads of all pathologies but that it may have an important influence on *human psycho-physical development depending, of course, on individual characteristics and on our quality of life*. In this way, it is possible to understand the features of mastication, its clinical implications, *its importance during development*, and, above all, the importance of choosing physiological treatment aimed at improving function during the age of growth and development.

Understanding and evaluation of function, in order to improve the important motor activity of mastication, represents a new and modern approach to creating a healthy stomatognathic system. To achieve this evolutionary dental/technical approach to true "curing" of the patient as a psycho-physical subject, it is necessary to abandon preconceptions of "not to worry, everything will adapt" and work toward a new concept of biological and physiological respect, based on neurological progress, of the unitariness of perception, action, and cognition. The choice of therapy will be influenced by the need to achieve a healthy and balanced stomatognathic system. The twentieth century was dominated essentially by the physiology of mandibular movement; in the twenty-first century, research has clearly shown the excellent discriminatory skill of the brain regarding dental inputs, confirmed by recent studies in fMRI (Toda and Taoka, 2001; Trulsson *et al.*, 2010), and the consequent, precise muscular activation. The road ahead is not easy – any change requires *mental flexibility* combined with a little *effort in order to acquire new skills, learning to reason and diagnose not only in terms of teeth, but, especially, of structural and functional equilibrium*, whilst having the skill and courage to choose *therapies that use dental assets to improve function*. Today, thanks to the results of research and efforts, all this is now finally possible. This book will explain the scientific results that prove the validity of this new approach, together with the biological/physiological actions and effects of the therapy. Understanding these concepts is fundamental from the outset, as is an open-minded approach to *considering teeth and their important receptor/neural features as a means (as opposed to an end) to achieve functional equilibrium*. This will allow us to understand *masticatory function – its clinical importance and effects on the stomatognathic system, the reasons why certain therapies improve it and others worsen it*, being careful not to reduce the study of mastication to a mere series of numbers that are statistically valid but of limited significance from a clinical point of view.

We will thus describe the general characteristics of the nervous and muscular systems, outlining them individually for didactic purposes, but never losing sight of the fact that they are in reality one and the same system. This book is not intended as a neurology textbook, but we will include a brief overview of the brain and its functions (comprehensible, we hope, also to non-specialized readers) where appropriate in order to explain the field of mastication.

3.2 The nervous system (Figures 3.2 and 3.3)

Both elementary forms of behavior and highly coordinated movements require intervention by the sensory, motor, and motivational systems. The function of the nervous system is based on three main functional systems:

- the *sensory system*, which collects peripheral information;
- the *motor system*, which activates and controls motor neurons;
- the *limbic system*, which acts on the motor system.

It is made up of:

- the *central nervous system*, which includes the brain and spinal cord.
- the *peripheral nervous system*, which includes ganglia and nerves outside the brain and spinal cord, divided into somatic and autonomic components.

The somatic component sends sensory signals regarding *muscle status*. Somatic motor neurons that innervate skeletal muscles, despite being classified as part of the peripheral nervous system, have their cellular body within the central nervous system, confirming the fact that these academic subdivisions are useful from a didactic point of view and for anatomical memorizing but that the achievement of function is characterized by the participation of the entire system without barriers or distinctions.

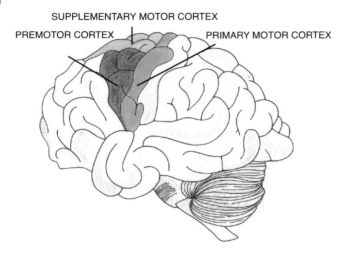

SUPPLEMENTARY MOTOR CORTEX

PREMOTOR CORTEX   PRIMARY MOTOR CORTEX

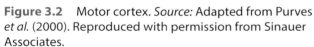

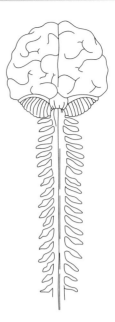

Figure 3.3 Spinal cord. *Source:* Adapted from Purves *et al.* (2000). Reproduced with permission from Sinauer Associates.

Figure 3.2 Motor cortex. *Source:* Adapted from Purves *et al.* (2000). Reproduced with permission from Sinauer Associates.

The autonomic component controls internal organs, smooth muscle fiber, and exocrine glands, and comprises:

- The sympathetic nervous system, responsible for stress control, may have an influence also on masticatory function. The change in proprioceptive information induced by an increase in sympathetic outflow has important implications, even under normal conditions, for the control of rhythmic motor function in states of high sympathetic activity (Roatta *et al.*, 2002, 2005).
- The parasympathetic nervous system, responsible for maintaining homeostasis.
- The enteric nervous system, which controls the smooth muscle fiber of the digestive system.

The structures that compose the central nervous system can be subdivided into

- the spinal cord;
- the medulla oblongata and the pons;
- the cerebellum;
- the mesencephalon (midbrain);
- the diencephalon (interbrain);
- the cortical and subcortical structures.

According to traditional anatomical classification, the medulla oblongata, pons, and mesencephalon comprise the brainstem. However, the pons and cerebellum share the same embryological origin and functional features (Kandel *et al.*, 2012).

3.2.1 The spinal cord (Figure 3.3)

The spinal cord *guarantees the mobility of the limbs*, and can autonomously perform a role of vital importance. It is 45 cm long and as thick as a pencil. It is characterized by a segmental-type form and consists of 31 pairs of spinal nerves.

The dorsal roots: these send data from muscles, skin and internal organs, and are characterized by the presence of paravertebral ganglia.

The ventral roots: these contain axons from motor neurons which innervate the muscles, sympathetic and parasympathetic pre-ganglionic axons.

3.2.2 Medulla oblongata and pons (Figure 3.4)

These connect the encephalon with the spinal cord and the brain with the cerebellum, maintaining the activity of the entire organ. They can be viewed as an extension of the spinal cord, dedicated to the cephalic area. They receive auditory and taste input and send data via the cranial nerves from the head, neck, and face. *They control autonomous and semi-autonomous activity* (blood pressure, heart rate, breathing, walking, etc.), *including mastication.*

Areas affecting mastication include the *trigeminal motor nucleus (central or rhythmic pattern generator) and the spinal trigeminal nucleus.* Both receive inputs from the periodontal mechanoreceptors.

3.2.3 The cerebellum (Figure 3.4)

The cerebellum plays an important role in motor control; it corrects errors, comparing the intention of movement with the reality and taking continuous action to correct faults. It is closely connected to the brainstem from functional and embryological points of view, and receives somatic-sensory afferents from the spinal cord and vestibular organs, and motor afferents from the cortex. Furthermore, it is involved in posture maintenance. It modulates the force and range of movement and is involved in learning motor skills. It coordinates movements and participates in motor cognitive processes, but in exactly what way is still not clear. Regarding mastication, it controls and corrects continuously masticatory movement with feedback-type mechanisms.

3.2.4 The mesencephalon (midbrain) (Figure 3.4)

This controls eye movement and skeletal muscles. It contains the nuclei for transmission of auditory and visual input.

Regarding mastication, it contains the trigeminal mesencephalic nucleus, which receives proprioceptive inputs of neuromuscular fuses and Golgi tendon organs, whether direct or crossed, from the masticatory muscles. This information is directed straight to the cerebellum, which performs a feedback-type motor control role as well as maintaining muscle tone, coordinating autonomous movements and subconscious balance. Furthermore, the trigeminal mesencephalic nucleus receives inputs from a limited number of mechanoreceptors in the periodontal ligament, which are then transmitted directly to the cerebellum, with the majority being organized with the aid of the Gasser ganglion (Byers and Dong, 1989; Nagata *et al.*, 2008).

Section 3.5, on automatisms of mastication, looks at this topic in more depth.

3.2.5 The diencephalon (Figure 3.4)

This is the home to retransmission of peripheral input to the cortex, and the control of hormonal secretions. Its central nucleus, *the thalamus, performs a gateway role providing access to consciousness, and is a compulsory relay station for all peripheral sensory information sent to the cortex.* It consists of:

• *The thalamus* – this processes all the sensory and motor input relayed to the cerebral cortex. It takes part in the maintenance of consciousness and emotions.

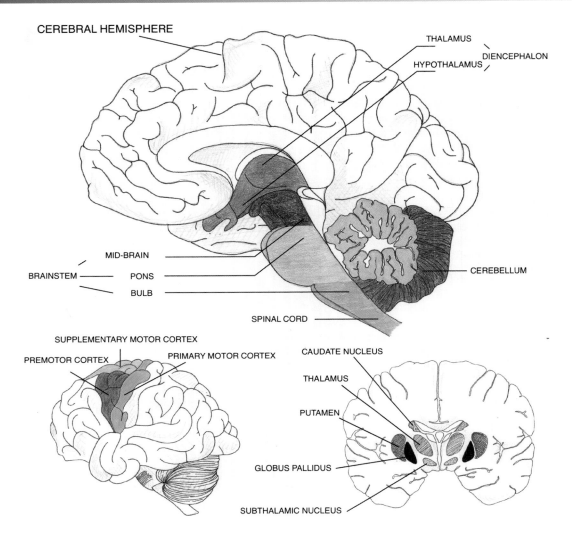

Figure 3.4 Central nervous system. *Source:* Adapted from Purves *et al.* (2000). Reproduced with permission from Sinauer Associates.

- *The hypothalamus* – this controls the autonomous nervous system and the secretion of hypophysis hormones. *It receives inputs from periodontal receptors* (Trulsson *et al.*, 2010).

3.2.6 **The cortical and subcortical structures** (Figure 3.4)

This constitutes approximately half or more of the human brain mass and hosts the integration of peripheral inputs, processing of motor responses, cognitive activity, consciousness, and more advanced mental processes that distinguish humans from animals. It comprises:

- The cerebral cortex, subdivided into four lobes (frontal, parietal, temporal, and occipital); it receives input from periodontal receptors.
- The white matter with basal ganglia (caudate, putamen, and globus pallidus), dedicated to motor control of mastication and rhythm (Masuda *et al.*, 2001).

- The hippocampus, involved in memory processes. Regarding mastication, the impairment of cognitive functions of selective attention and recognition memory in the prefrontal cortex and hippocampus were recorded in mice with altered mastication due to premature extraction (during development) of molar teeth (Johnston *et al.*, 2012; Kawahata *et al.*, 2014).

  Studies on human subjects with fMRI have shown that, during chewing, the reaction time significantly decreases and that increased activation occurs in the anterior cingulate cortex, left frontal gyrus for the executive network, and motor-related regions for both attentional networks (Takada and Miyamoto, 2004; Hirano *et al.*, 2013).

  Studies on older subjects have shown that low chewing ability is associated with lower cognitive functioning, depression, and food insufficiency. Whether elderly people chew with natural dentition or prostheses does not make a difference: the chewing ability contributes significantly to the preservation of cognitive abilities. The results add to the evidence of the association between chewing ability and cognitive impairment (as well as cognitive dysfunction) in the elderly (Weijenberg *et al.*, 2011).

- The amygdala, responsible for controlling emotions (Purves *et al.*, 2009; Kandel *et al.*, 2012).

3.3 Receptors in the stomatognathic system (Figure 3.5)

The central nervous system receives signals from the peripheral receptors via the brainstem, thalamus, and cerebral cortex. The quantity and quality of data sent to the brain depends on the characteristics of the receptors and their concentration. The speed with which this information is sent to the brain depends on the type of neural connection.

Regarding the stomatognathic system, we know that the *receptors are deeply concentrated, highly specialized, and connected to the central nervous system also by electrical synapses*, which transmit inputs with high speed. This means that any change within the stomatognathic system is immediately perceived by the central nervous system with extreme precision. We know for certain that mammals' teeth (including human teeth) have highly refined discriminatory powers. This applies to control of functional movements such as deglutition, mastication, and so on, whilst any therapeutic, orthodontic, prosthetic, or conservative therapy will be immediately registered by the brain, which then adjusts/compensates functional movement via control of the masticatory muscles. *A thorough understanding of the characteristics of the receptors in the stomatognathic system is therefore vital for any dentist, irrespective of their specialization.*

Thus, we will give a brief overview of the topic.

The receptors of the stomatognathic system are located in the oral mucous membrane, tongue, teeth, and periodontal and TMJ and muscles. They are numerous receptors (more highly concentrated in certain areas), sensitive (low threshold; i.e., they respond even to very weak stimuli) and specialized (sensitive to the direction and target direction of applied forces). We will look deeply at periodontal mechanoreceptors because these are the ones directly involved in the dental field and in the motor control of mastication. However, the mucous membrane and tongue receptors, transporting taste and tactile data, are also of importance. On the basis of this information concerning consistency, taste, dimensions, and bolus position, the cortex then processes and establishes the type of chewing cycle most suitable for the grinding of the food in question, checking and adjusting to bolus changes throughout mastication. *These receptors play a precise role in motor control of chewing patterns* and follow neural paths similar to those of mechanoreceptors, in the oral mucus and tongue (Morquette *et al.*, 2012) (Figure 3.6).

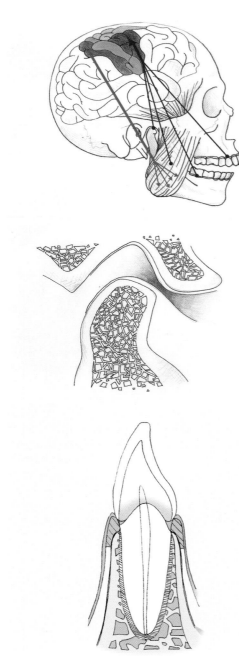

Figure 3.5 Peripheral receptors of the stomatognathic system. *Source:* Adapted from Purves *et al.* (2000). Reproduced with permission from Sinauer Associates.

3.3.1 Receptors of the temporomandibular joint

These are *low-threshold receptors, extremely sensitive and specialized*, which are innervated by the auriculotemporal nerve. They are *more highly concentrated in the lateral and posterior areas of the articular capsule*, whilst the anterior part, comprising the meniscus and synovial membrane, contains few or no receptors.

Various types of receptors in the TMJ with differing characteristics have been identified:

- Pacinian corpuscles, characterized by *rapid adjustment*. They signal the beginning and end of the movement, as well as controlling it. They activate simultaneously during mandibular movement.
- Ruffini's endings, *which do not adjust*. These provide information on condyle and mandibular posture. They are highly sensitive – each receptor activates according to a precise opening angle of the mouth. They discharge continuously.
- Golgi's corpuscles, featuring limited adjustment capacity. These are activated by intense pressure and play a protective role.
- Free nerve endings, which transmit nociceptor stimuli.

The characteristics of receptors in the TMJ allow us to reproduce mandibular position in space without physical references. The sensory information transmitted by the TMJ *receptors codifies the position, shifting and speed of condylar movement, within a physiological shift of the mandible during the opening movement* (Tsuboi *et al.*, 2009). More specifically, *they play an important role in sending sensory information regarding condyle movement*, particularly during the opening stage of the chewing cycle (Morquette *et al.*, 2012).

The maturation of temporomandibular receptors occurs at an early stage of masticatory development, and their function is linked to the joint load established during mastication. According to diet consistency, the articular receptors become more or less active, maintaining their relatively short recovery time as a result of a diet without joint load (Ishida *et al.*, 2013). This *direct relationship* between development, activity of joint receptors, and masticatory function is of great clinical importance as it *proves how function*

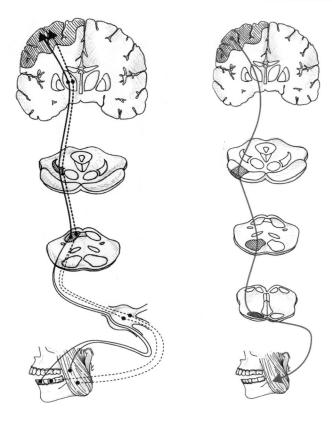

Figure 3.6   Peripheral inputs and central output.

is related to histological and biomolecular issues of tissues. Knowing that the *receptors are formed and modulate their activity according to function*, it is easy to see how important diet, teeth, and occlusion are as a factor in harmonious growth of the TMJ.

This is particularly true if we consider that at birth the TMJ is completely undeveloped and, on the basis of histological studies (Thilander *et al.*, 1976), its growth is of an adaptive type. Therefore, all dental therapies may influence (at greater or lesser levels) the TMJ function and development, with orthodontic therapies being among the most important.

3.3.2 Periodontal mechanoreceptors (Figure 3.7)

These are *highly sensitive and specialized receptors* directly involved in the dental field. It is necessary to know their features in order to understand the influence of occlusion and dental inputs on neuromuscular motor control of mastication. For this reason we will describe them in depth. Periodontal receptors have been analyzed *with histological and electrophysiological studies, but not always with concordant results.*

Periodontal mechanoreceptors are known to be receptors in the periodontal ligament that respond to surprisingly low contact force levels (<1 N) applied to the teeth. The functions of nerve fibers in the periodontal ligament, junctional epithelium, and gingiva are coordinated with the dental pulp and dentin innervation to form an integrated set of sensory systems needed for normal somatosensory reflexes and perception of the external forces on teeth. Their ultrastructural specialization is related to the functional properties of the periodontal innervation (threshold, adaptation, etc.).

Although various kinds of mechanoreceptors are present in the periodontal ligament, studies have shown that the Ruffini ending is the primary mechanoreceptor in this location (Byers, 1985). The Ruffini endings are usually distributed in specialized compartments of dense connective tissue, such as tendons, the fibrous part of joints and ligaments, or around hairs (Andres and Von During, 1973); they have been categorized as low-threshold, stretch mechanoreceptors of slowly adapting type II (Chambers *et al.*, 1972; Biemesdefer *et al.*, 1978) and comprise multiple-branching nerve fibers encapsulated in thin connective-tissue membranes; *the periodontal mechanoreceptors are slowly adapting, direction sensitive, low-threshold stretch receptors of Ruffini type. They do not usually show any capsule around the endings* and are characterized by specialized finger-like structures extending out from the terminals into the extracellular matrix of the ligament; this may offer more rapidly adapting properties in the periodontium than the capsulated cylindrical receptors in the skin (Byers, 1985; Dong *et al.*, 1993).

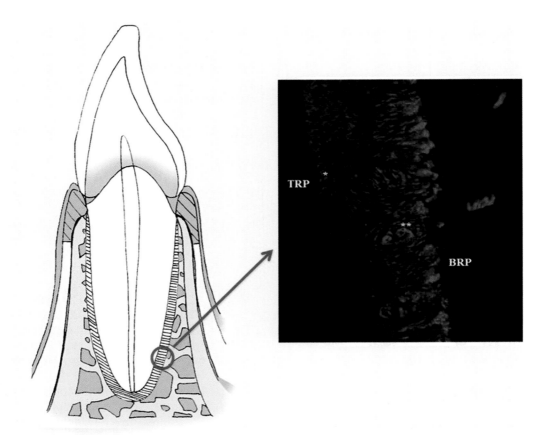

Figure 3.7 Immunofluorescence reaction for PGP 9.5 in periodontal ligament of rat incisor. It is possible to observe a low PGP 9.5 immunostaining (red fluorescence) in the tooth-related part (TRP*), where it marks thin lines of nervous fibers; instead, in the bone-related part (BRP**) it is possible to observe a high PGP 9.5 immunofluorescence pattern that marks, prevalently, receptor endings of nervous fibers. *Source:* G. Anastasi and G. Cutroneo, University of Messina, Messina, Italy. Reproduced with permission from G. Anastasi and G. Cutroneo.

The main periodontal Ruffini nerve endings have been classified as types 1 and 2. Type 1 shows lamellar terminal Schwann cells and expanded axon terminals with axonal spines that penetrate surrounding tissue; type 2 is characterized by lesser-branched Ruffini endings with fewer axonal spines, less basal lamina, and fewer Schwann cells. Both of these receptor types are present in the periodontal ligament (Maeda *et al.*, 1999). The amount of receptoplasm is higher in the periodontal Ruffini endings receptors than in the high-threshold nociceptors (Byers and Maeda, 1997).

The fibers are associated with Schwann cells (termed lamellar or terminal Schwann cells), which possess kidney-shaped nuclei (K-cells) and share many ultrastructural features with support cells of other mechanoreceptive terminals such as Meissner or Pacinian corpuscles. The characteristics of the Schwann cells and their relative adjacent nerve fibers are fundamental to understanding the behavior of periodontal Ruffini mechanoreceptors. The developmental responses of periodontal Ruffini mechanoreceptors depend on molecular mechanisms located in Schwann lamellae and not on axonal mechanisms (Byers and Maeda, 1997).

Periodontal mechanoreceptors are *concentrated in the bone alveolus-related part of the ligament* (Ochi *et al.*, 1997), *in the regions subjected to stretch during tooth use* (Figure 3.7); their location can change during development and aging. Different types of teeth show a different distribution of receptors depending on tooth shape and function (Byers and Maeda, 1997). Ruffini mechanoreceptors are contained in the interdental ligaments also, being likely involved in detecting movements of one tooth relative to another. The mechanoreceptors arborize primarily in the dense portion of the ligament, less in the loose perivascular region. The largest endings occur near the apex of the root for most teeth, but on the lingual side of rodent incisors (that are continuously erupting teeth) (Byers and Maeda, 1997).

The mechanoreceptors have been studied not only from a histological point of view, but also with electrophysiological experiments. Since these studies, the mechanoreceptors have been classified as "slowly" and "rapidly" adapting receptors, but, unfortunately, they are not clearly related to a specific histological type of nerve ending. A type 3 ending with coiled form (similar to a rapidly adapting Meissner corpuscle) may represent a rapidly adapting form.

The cutaneous Ruffini endings are of slowly adaptive type only. From the functional data of Cash and Linden, the most slowly adapting receptors were located at the apex of the tooth, while the rapidly adapting receptors were located close to the fulcrum of the tooth (Cash and Linden, 1982; Linden and Scott, 1989), but the authors suggest that there might be only one type of periodontal mechanoreceptor adapting to the different functional demands. This important issue is still not clear, because the results are deductive and remain unconfirmed by histological evaluation.

From animal studies, the threshold sufficient to evoke a response from the majority of the slowly adapting units was between 0.01 and 0.05 N (Cash and Linden, 1982; Johnsen and Trulsson, 2003; Nagata *et al.*, 2008). Displacements of the tooth in the order of 2–3 μm would seem to be sufficient to evoke a response in single neurons. A critical amount of the stimulus is necessary to elicit a response from the rapidly adapting unit, and the latency of response decreases as the application of the stimulus is increased. *The mechanoreceptors are very sensitive to the stimulus direction.* The optimal stimulus directions of the incisor-sensitive neurons of rats are oriented labio-lingually or linguo-labially (Tabata and Hayashi, 1994). Subsequent electrophysiological studies on the trigeminal ganglion of rats have shown that in the maxillary molar-sensitive units the orientation of the predominant optimal stimulus direction was linguo-buccal or bucco-lingual. In the mandibular molar-sensitive units, the optimal stimulus direction was linguo-buccal, and the units were excited by stimulation of the buccal cusp. *Interestingly, the optimal directions are those useful in chewing food* (Tabata *et al.*, 2002, 2006) (Figure 3.8).

Regarding slow and rapid receptors, the same authors showed that *they are located differently in upper and lower molars*, with the rapid receptors being more represented in the mandibular teeth (which convey the information from the mandible; i.e., the moving bone) and the slow adapting receptors in the maxillary molars. The differentiation between upper and lower teeth, and between anterior and posterior teeth, is important because of their different functional role (Tabata *et al.*, 2006).

Also, changes during development and load response reflect *the strict relationship between function and periodontal mechanoreceptors maturation. One of the greatest changes during development in the stomatognathic system is the functional conversion of feeding behavior from sucking to chewing* (Barlow, 2009). Since functional conversion is related to the development and maturation of the peripheral nervous system, a number of interesting developmental studies have demonstrated that *the morpho-physiological maturation of periodontal Ruffini endings is closely related to the tooth eruption* (Asahito *et al.*, 1999) and that *the final arborization of the Ruffini*

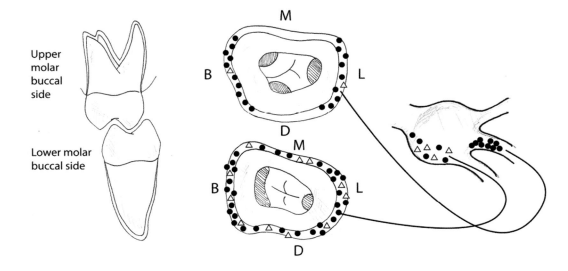

Upper molar buccal side

Lower molar buccal side

Figure 3.8 Different characteristics of the upper and lower molar periodontal mechanoreceptors in experimental studies in rats. Interestingly, the rapid-adapting receptors (black triangles) are more concentrated in the lower molars, which convey information from the moving bone, and the slow-adapting receptors are more concentrated in the maxillary molars. B: buccal; M: mesial; L: lingual; D: distal. *Source:* Tabata *et al.* (2006). Reproduced with permission from Elsevier.

endings, of axonal spines, and thickening of basement membrane are completed shortly after the beginning of the function of rat incisors (Nakakura-Ohshima *et al.*, 1995; Hayashi *et al.*, 2000) or molar function (Umemura *et al.*, 2010).

Interestingly, in this last study, *no difference was displayed for the neurons conveying the inputs of the muscle spindle of the masticatory muscles after tooth eruption*. This is due to the fact that these neurons have been active since the embryonic period, as swallowing starts in utero.

Various studies have shown that multiple neurotrophins, such as glial-cell-line-derived neurotrophic factor, and Schwann cells are fundamental and stage specific for the maturation and maintenance of the periodontal Ruffini endings. These neurotrophins are also important because they mediate trophic effects on neuronal survival, growth, and target innervation (Hayashi *et al.*, 2000; Hoshino *et al.*, 2003; Maruyama *et al.*, 2005; Igarashi *et al.*, 2007; Ohishi *et al.*, 2009).

Periodontal mechanoreceptors are directly involved in the response to occlusal load. Sodeyama *et al.* (1996) demonstrated on rats, with different occlusal forces, that *occlusal trauma induces specific changes in the distribution and shape of nerve terminals in the periodontal ligament*; other studies on rats showed that an improper occlusal force reversibly alters both the axon terminals (Shi *et al.*, 2006) and the functional properties of the periodontal Ruffini endings (Asano *et al.*, 2007).

The results of many studies in humans and animals, recording the electrophysiological activity from periodontal mechanoreceptors, have demonstrated the presence of two basic receptor types, both of which respond to teeth movements following the application of an external force. One type is the rapid adapting unit: this generates transient discharges to a sustained stimulus, and the number of impulses produced is dependent on the rate of application of the stimulus; at faster application rates, more neural impulses are produced. Thus, they are sensitive to both the rate and magnitude of the applied load, but respond only when the load is being applied (Hannam, 1982).

The slowly adapting unit, unlike the other type of unit, continues to generate nerve impulses for longer periods, throughout the tooth displacement and even when the load is no longer exerted on the tooth. In this type of receptor, the frequency of the impulse during the initiation of the response increases with increased stimulus; the initial and final frequencies are also dependent on the magnitude of the applied load (Hannam, 1982; Trulsson and Essick, 2010).

The results strongly suggest that *periodontal mechanoreceptors play a significant role in the specification of the forces used to hold and manipulate food between teeth*, and in these respects the masticatory system appears analogous to fine finger-control mechanisms used during precision manipulation of small objects (Nishino *et al.*, 1991; Ishii *et al.*, 2002; Trulsson *et al.*, 2010).

3.3.3 Muscular receptors (Figure 3.9)
Muscle receptors comprise the following:

- Muscle spindles, which are encapsulated sensory receptors with a fusiform shape located in the muscle. They provide information on muscle length. In the masseter, there are many more of these than there are muscle fibers. The structure and functional behavior of muscle spindle is very complex, allowing a refined neuromuscular control (Purves *et al.*, 2009).

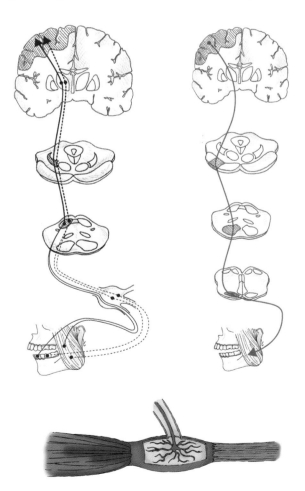

Figure 3.9   Muscular receptors and motor control.

- Golgi tendon organs, which are sensory receptors located at the junction between the fiber muscles and tendon. They provide information on the changes in muscle tension. The firing frequency of these receptors gives a fairly accurate estimate of the total force in a contracting muscle.
- Extrafusal receptors, which perceive harmful stimuli.

The cellular body of the afferent neuron is located in the trigeminal mesencephalic nucleus, where it contracts synapses with the second neuron connected to the cerebellum (see Section 3.2.4, the trigeminal mesencephalic nucleus).

The motor plaques, in the masseter muscle, control just a few fibers (contrary to the muscles of limbs), which allows an extremely precise control of the muscular contraction. This can be easily modified during muscular activity in order to adapt the chewing pattern to the functional requirements.

3.4 Reflex movements

Reflex is an involuntary movement, caused by the application of a necessary stimulus, whose anatomical foundation is a reflex arc comprising two or more neurons (interneurons). Reflex movements do not change with use.

Generally, reflexes are characterized by a stimulant component in a group of agonist muscles and an inhibitory component in an antagonist group.

On the contrary, *masticatory muscles are characterized by an important stimulant component of closing muscles (agonist) and a weak inhibitory component of opening muscles (antagonist)*. This phenomenon is backed up by a large number of receptors in the closing muscles (agonist) and a small number of receptors in opening muscles (antagonist) (Woda, 1984). We know that mastication is supported by continuous, autonomous, and controlled force movements; however, some reflexes can be evoked in the stomatognathic system on the basis of suitable stimuli.

3.4.1 Closing reflexes (comparable to spinal extensor reflexes)

These are achieved with up–down percussion of the chin, which stretches the elevator muscles and then stimulates the neuromuscular fuses of the same muscles. As opposed to spinal reflexes which are characterized by inhibition of antagonist muscles, in the stomatognathic system, *inhibition of the depressor muscles is minimal*. This reflex is a jaw jerk/masseter reflex or trigeminal myotatic reflex which lifts the mandible (Woda, 1984).

3.4.2 Opening reflexes (comparable to spinal flexor reflexes)

These are characterized *by stimulation of depressor muscles and inhibition of elevator muscles*. Nociceptor stimuli have their own paths in the cephalic area too, just as in the rest of the body. Differently from spinal reflexes, however, contraction of depressors and inhibition of elevators in the cephalic area is *bilateral*. The stimulant component (stimulation of depressors) does not exist in humans but manifests in silent periods. *The opening of the mandible is therefore a consequence of inhibited elevators rather than stimulated depressors*, with two silent periods corresponding to the inhibitory component of the non-nociceptor reflex and that of the nociceptor reflex. The lowering of the mandible appears a result of gravity force (Woda, 1984; Aigouy et al., 1988).

3.4.2.1 Non-nociceptor opening reflex

In all reflexes, the stimulant component of a group of agonist muscles is connected with the inhibitory component of a group of antagonist muscles; in this case, the depressor and elevator muscles of the mandible.

Owing to the different strengths of the two muscle groups involved, *the inhibitory component of opening reflex of the mouth is extremely important*, to the point that there is a group of interneurons that forms the "supratrigeminal" nucleus, dedicated to the inhibition of elevator muscles. The mechanical stimulation of dental, periodontal, lingual mucus, palatal, and TMJ receptors provokes the *inhibition of elevator muscles*. The paths of the two components are disynaptic.

3.4.2.2 Nociceptor opening reflex

This provides *protection from nociceptor stimuli*, such as biting of the tongue. It is activated by stimulation of the oral–facial mucous membrane, pulp, TMJ, and periodontium. The paths of the stimulating and inhibitory components are polysynaptic (Woda, 1984).

3.5 **Automatic movements** (Figures 3.10 and 3.11)

For any voluntary motor action to take place it is necessary for the movement to be planned, performed, and then constantly controlled/corrected with the aid of integrated postural adjustments. If (as in the case of mastication) the movement is rhythmic and managed by brain automatisms, motor control is even more complex and involves the entire brain. Above all, we must bear in mind before tackling neural control of mastication that the work of the brain, perception, and action is a single, unitary process. For didactic reasons and clarity, we will talk about afferent and efferent pathways, hierarchies, and sequentiality. But the result is much more than the sum of single parts. Many of the single elements have been discovered, but many more elements of the "overall complex" remain yet to be revealed and understood. One of these aspects is, certainly, the influence or interaction of the limbic system with the motor system which, in humans, interests the more recently acquired associative areas of thought and that, in the case of mastication, is clearly involved. We know that eating, nowadays, is much more a question of satisfaction than a question of survival and aggression. These aspects will not be considered in this book being dedicated to the relationship between occlusion and function, but an adolescent at risk of eating disorder should be diagnosed before any orthodontic therapy.

Automatic movements are genetically preprogrammed mechanisms that are modified by exercises and experience. Their efficiency improves with use. They are very different from reflexes, which are stereotyped involuntary movements and do not alter with use.

What role can these definitions play in the daily work of a professional orthodontist or dentist? Knowledge and understanding of these mechanisms allow us to comprehend the positive or negative effects of occlusion/malocclusion on function. To be more specific: *as they are "genetically pre-programmed," automatisms are inherited by the child and will be modified on the basis of peripheral information*. This happens for the rhythmic motor actions that take place with a refined and continuous interaction between genetics and environment, especially in the first 3 years of life. *Amongst the various movements to be mastered* (walking, running, jumping, etc.), *there is also mastication*, where the motor pattern is adapted according to peripheral inputs.

The primary motor cortex may be involved predominantly in the initiation and control of jaw movements, and the ventral premotor cortex may be involved in motor preparation, playing a role as a higher order motor area related to the initiation and control of jaw movements. These areas, which are the ventrolateral portion of Brodmann's areas four and six, are called the "cortical mastication areas" (Bracco *et al.*, 2010). As mastication is a rhythmic, semi-automatic activity, it is supported by autofiring cells, located in the nuclei of the base and in the brainstem (Dellow and Lund, 1971). The first group of neurons involved in the automatism of mastication is located in the

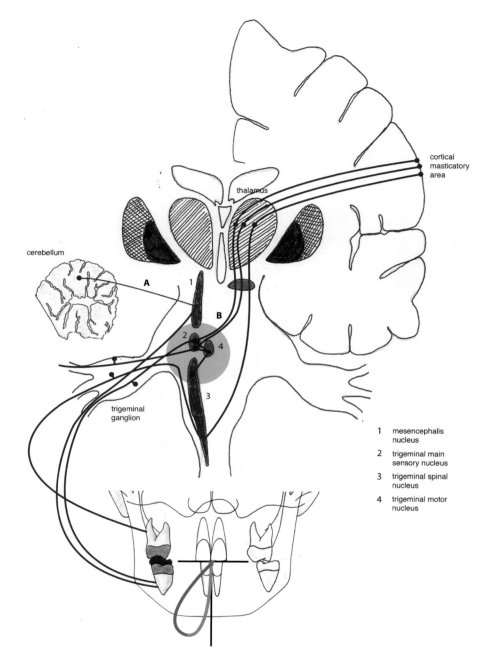

Figure 3.10 The inputs arising from the periodontal mechanoreceptors of teeth have a powerful influence on the motor control.

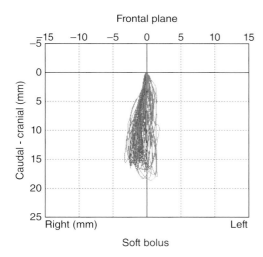

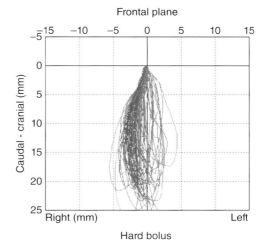

Figure 3.11 Continuous adaptability of the chewing pattern to the bolus type during chewing on the right side.

brainstem between the pons and medulla oblongata and is called the "central pattern generator." Following the discovery of the central pattern generator, other groups of autofiring neurons involved in the automatism of masticatory function were identified in the basal ganglia. The central pattern generator, also called the rhythmic pattern generator, is represented as an area, rather than a nucleus, which may directly receive the inputs from mechanoreceptors (Figure 3.12).

The motor cortex is connected to the *spinal trigeminal nucleus and the rhythmic pattern generator located in the brainstem*. These two complexes are, respectively, the nucleus, which receives *sensory afferents, and the generator, responsible for maintaining masticatory rhythm*.

The *spinal trigeminal nucleus* receives most of the information from the periodontal mechano-receptors, via the central extension of "T" *cells in the Gasserian ganglion*. In the spinal trigeminal nucleus, the central extension of "T" neurons of the Gasserian ganglion contracts synapses with the second sensory neuron of the nucleus, and from here the *axons of the second neuron* set off upward to the thalamus (via the trigeminal lemniscus) where the third sensory neuron is located, which then goes to the cortex. However, some studies have identified sensory fibers that arrive directly at the cortex.

A significant finding for the comprehension of motor control of mastication is that inputs departing from periodontal dental mechanoreceptors not only arrive at *the trigeminal sensory nucleus but are also able to activate the trigeminal motor nucleus*, thus directly influencing the chewing motor control.

Recent research has underlined the significance of feedback from periodontal input to the rhythmic pattern generator in the brainstem during chewing (Morquette *et al.*, 2012). The afferent neurons in the trigeminal ganglion are active during mastication when using the molar teeth, especially during the power phase of closure, and are sensitive to the force (or changes of force) applied to the tooth. A model has recently been proposed in which sensory feedback might be responsible for the regulation, through astrocyte activation, of the bursting pattern and frequency of the rhythm generator population of the rhythmic pattern generator (Morquette *et al.*, 2012).

Peripheral and cortical inputs from the cortical masticatory area contribute, synergistically, to a more efficient astrocytic activation, decreasing the extracellular Ca^{2+} and enhancing the

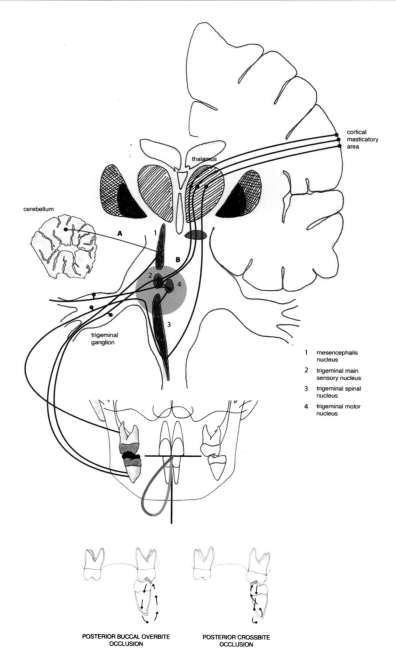

cortical
masticatory
area

thalamus

cerebellum

A

B

1

2

4

3

trigeminal
ganglion

1 mesencephalis
   nucleus

2 trigeminal main
   sensory nucleus

3 trigeminal spinal
   nucleus

4 trigeminal motor
   nucleus

POSTERIOR BUCCAL OVERBITE
OCCLUSION

POSTERIOR CROSSBITE
OCCLUSION

Figure 3.12 The motor control adapts to the peripheral inputs from the mechanoreceptors of teeth, which are influenced by occlusion and malocclusions.

sodium current. This could, momentarily, turn the population of neurons into the rhythm generator's driving premotoneurons or motoneurons directly. The bursting pattern and frequency of this population could be adjusted by sensory feedback since sensory fibers provide depolarizing inputs activating the bursting neurons (Morquette *et al.*, 2012). *The powerful influence of the periodontal mechanoreceptors on the central pattern generator* has been clearly demonstrated in experimental studies (Morimoto *et al.*, 1984; Lund *et al.*, 1999; Lund and Kolta, 2006). It is interesting to note that the mechanism underlying the adaptive processes of movement consists of changes to the neural structure. In particular, the peripheral information is very efficient at programming and establishing motor memory. This explains how nociceptor stimuli from teeth (conscious or not) such as cusp-to-cusp contacts caused by malocclusion, *whether in deciduous or permanent dentition, have a significant influence on the development of chewing pattern motor memory (Figure 3.12). The earlier the peripheral input arises, the earlier the pattern will be established, as, for example, happens in unilateral posterior crossbite.* This malocclusion is established during the early stages of a child's development, deeply influencing the motor pattern of mastication. Control and compensatory adjustment of movement (for mastication) is very important because the chewing pattern adjusts to peripheral input, particularly from the periodontal mechanoreceptors, which have a strong influence on the occlusal phase of closure for bolus grinding. *In the early stages of development, the system adapts for optimal function.*

Much remains still to be discovered regarding the characteristics of human mechanoreceptors, in light of the fact that research into the stomatognathic system is constrained by the differences between laboratory animals and humans. However, the influence of dental inputs on the refined sensory–motor–cognitive–emotive control in humans is nowadays undeniable (Trulsson *et al.*, 2010).

3.6 Motor control: feedback and feed-forward (Figures 3.13 and 3.14)

Movement is constantly controlled by feedback compensatory mechanisms and feed-forward anticipatory mechanisms.

Feedback compensatory mechanisms are supported by the brainstem circuits, the cerebellum, and the basal nuclei, which are connected with the cerebral cortex. In particular, the cerebellum is an "error corrector," in the sense that it compares the idea of the movement with the actual reality and then, continuously, corrects it.

Feed-forward anticipatory mechanisms are instead under the control of the cerebral cortex, reacting according to cutaneous, visual and sensory stimuli. In other words, the movement is predicted and the muscle involved is activated even before the movement itself begins. Feed-forward mechanisms have been identified also in the masseter (Komuro *et al.*, 2001).

To sum up, neural control of mastication involves:

- the cerebral cortex, which plans and programs the chewing pattern according to bolus type and peripheral inputs;
- the brainstem, cerebellum, and basal nuclei, which maintain rhythm and regulate chewing pattern.

The cerebellum, brainstem, basal nuclei, and cortex all continually regulate movement with anticipatory and compensatory mechanisms.

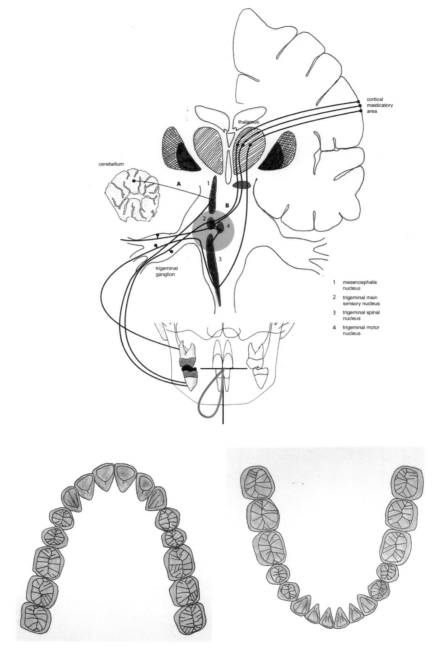

Figure 3.13 The inputs arising from the periodontal mechanoreceptors of teeth, especially from the posterior region of the occlusion, have a powerful influence on the motor control of chewing.

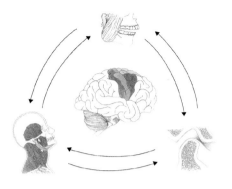

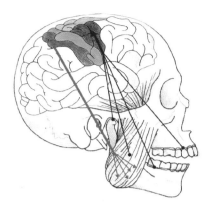

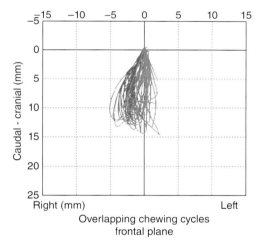

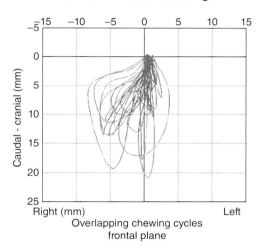

Figure 3.14   The motor control adapts the chewing pattern to the peripheral inputs. Top left: *Source for the muscles:* Redrawn from Neff (1999). *Source for the brain:* Redrawn from Purves *et al.* (2000). Reproduced with permission of Sinauer Associates.

3.7 **Neuromuscular control** (Figure 3.15)

In this section we will look at neuromuscular control of masticatory muscles during mastication. This is a complex issue that regards neural control (i.e. refined over time), and has been the subject of very few heterogeneous studies. This is probably due to the difficulty of such research, both regarding the selection and classification of samples (which requires clinical experience and skills in order to avoid bias) and regarding the aspect of equipment (which requires suitable technologies and specific software programs). This type of research calls for multidisciplinary skills and collaborations.

On the contrary, there are numerous works on masticatory muscle during *maximum clenching*. It is of importance to underline that these two types of studies, maximum clenching and

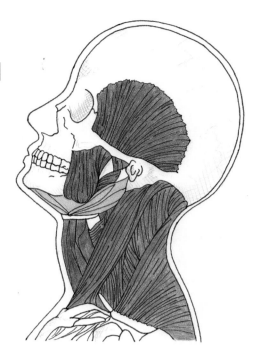

Figure 3.15 Representation of different groups of muscles of head and neck in different colors. *Source:* Redrawn and adapted from Neff (1999).

mastication, are deeply different and not comparable. Muscle activity during maximum clenching displays features similar to those of *a border movement*, whilst *muscle activity during mastication is a rhythmic movement coordinated between sides.* The former is a voluntary movement that involves muscles of the two sides in an optimal, symmetric, and simultaneous manner. The latter is, instead, a semi-automatic movement that requires coordination between the two sides which are physiologically involved in an asymmetric way during the execution of each single chewing cycle. The general symmetry of the system during chewing depends on the alternation of mastication between the two sides. Obviously, when such alternation is lost (for any reason) then unilateral mastication (or predominantly unilateral) determines functional asymmetry. This concept will be examined in depth later. We will not analyze the technical characteristics of electromyography acquisition in this book, but we advise the interested readers to consult the works of specialized bioengineers on the topic (Merletti, 1999, 2000; Merlo *et al.*, 2003; Farina and Merletti, 2003; Merlo and Campanini, 2010). We will instead look more in depth at the neuromuscular and clinical characteristics of masticatory muscles to understand masticatory function and the clinical, diagnostic, and therapeutic aspects of malocclusions.

3.7.1 General characteristics of masticatory muscles

Jaw muscles are active during a large variety of motor tasks, such as mastication, biting, speech, and swallowing. To execute this variety of tasks they must be able to control the position of the mandible precisely, and instantaneously apply changing forces to it. The jaw muscles can meet these different requirements because of their complex and particular architecture, which, in combination with a heterogeneous composition of fibers, is capable of producing a variety of forces at different contraction speeds (Korfage *et al.*, 2005).

We previously described that in neural control of mastication the cortex is organized in "cortical columns" that control not just one but a group of muscles in the role of performing a specific movement. In a similar way, muscles are currently classified in groups, characterized by the same embryogenetic origins and their shared contribution toward performing the same movement.

Masticatory muscles, therefore, must be considered as a "group of muscles" that work together in a synergetic and coordinated way, especially during the closure stage of mastication. They are called *"elevator muscles"* and correspond to the antigravity extensor and posture muscles of the rest of the body. These are very powerful muscles characterized by a high concentration of receptors and subject to precise neural control. The group of masticatory muscles that work to raise the mandible (closing) comprises: the anterior temporalis, the masseter, the medial pterygoid, and the lateral pterygoid.

Suprahyoid muscles are a group of muscles dedicated to mouth opening and defined as *"depressor muscles."* They correspond to flexor muscles in the rest of the body but, as already stated, have a low concentration of receptors.

The group of suprahyoid muscles that work to lower the mandible (opening) comprises: biventer or digastric, stylo-hyoideus, mylo-hyoideus, and genio-hyoideus.

The group of infrahyoid muscles that work to depress and stabilize the hyoid bone comprises: sterno-hyoideus, sterno-thyroideus, thyroideus, and homo-hyoideus.

The group of neck muscles is represented by the trapezius, sternocleidomastoid, and the intrinsic neck muscles (Neff, 1999).

The precision with which masticatory muscles are controlled by the central nervous system suggests that these muscles have particular macroscopic and microscopic characteristics. From a macroscopic point of view the masseter displays a feathered or semi-feathered arrangement characterized by the presence of an aponeurosis. The aponeurosis is made up of collagen fiber, such as tendons, and has bands of bone between the zygomatic arch and the external face of the mandibular angle. Muscle fibers within the aponeurosis may be short and numerous (increasing of maximum force). This arrangement allows *the development of a wider force. Furthermore, the independent status of each band allows a different action to be executed, rendering the muscle easily adaptable to neuromuscular control and able to respond with high precision*. In the case of the masseter the functional unit is the aponeurosis band, rather than the muscle.

The cell body of neurons that transport the proprioceptive afferents of elevator muscles of the mandible via the fifth pair of cranial nerves (the trigeminal) is found in the mesencephalic nucleus of the trigeminal in the brainstem of the central nervous system, connected to the cerebellum and the neural pattern of unconscious reflexes. An important feature is the presence of electrical synapses in addition to chemical synapses, which allows quicker and more powerful muscle contraction. Furthermore, the number of fibers per motor unit is very low, indicating highly precise neural control and high capacities of response and adjustment.

3.7.2 Microscopic characteristics of masticatory muscles

Compared with limb and trunk muscles, the jaw muscles are highly unusual.

Masticatory muscles, particularly the masseters, are characterized by rapidly and slowly contracting fibers. But, in addition to normal slow type I and fast type II fibers, many of the fibers are hybrid. Another remarkable feature is the fact that they contain fiber types that are typical for developing or cardiac muscle (Korfage *et al.*, 2005).

Type I are red muscle fibers with slow contraction and are characterized by:

- long-lasting contractions and low intensity;
- aerobic glycolysis;
- high resistance to fatigue;
- high capillary spread;
- inferior diameter compared with rapid fibers;
- high concentration of mitochondrial content and oxidative enzymes;
- high concentration of myoglobin;
- typical of muscles allocated to the maintenance of posture or muscles that produce slow and repetitive movements.

Type IIA are red intermediary muscle fibers with rapid contraction and display:

- rapid contraction, although less rapid than white fibers;
- less fatigue than white muscle fibers;
- a good recovery capacity;
- a good quantity of myosin;

- both aerobic and anaerobic capacity;
- response to training.

Type IIB are white muscle fibers with rapid contraction and are characterized by:

- short bursts of maximum power;
- an anaerobic (low-performance) pathway;
- hydrolyzing adenosine triphosphate extremely quickly and producing quick contraction of the sarcomere;
- easy fatigue;
- limited capillary spread;
- low content of myoglobin and mitochondria;
- responding to alpha phasic motor neurons with high-speed contraction;
- high levels of glycogen;
- grouping in smaller numbers within a motor unit;
- development of increased power and adjustment to brief bursts of effort.

Type II X fast fibers are resistant to fatigue (between type IIA and IIB).

The structures of masticatory muscles and connections with the central nervous system are programmed to send information and regulate neuromuscular response in an extremely rapid and precise way.

Hybrid fiber types, in limb and trunk muscles, are thought to be those in transition from one fiber type to another. Hybrid fibers are abundantly present in normal jaw-closing muscle, both in rabbits and in humans. The important presence of hybrid fibers in considerable numbers may be due to specific functional demands of the masseter muscle; these fiber types probably increase the capacity of the masseter muscle to generate a large variety of motor tasks, since they have contractile features that lie between those of pure fibers.

In this way, the presence of *hybrid fibers could reflect the adaptive ability of masseter muscle fibers, showing the capacity to modify their contractile properties to optimize the efficiency during contraction*. Then, the masseter muscle could continuously switch from one fiber type to another. Based on its functional demand, these continuous changes in phenotypic structures could also influence normal arrangement of the entire muscle.

Since *masseter muscle* is subject to continuous mechanical stress, as a result of continuous control of the position and motion of the mandible and creation of forces at the teeth and TMJ level, *this muscle is characterized by a particular high turnover, which produces a regeneration process initiated by fibers typical of developing muscle*. A further remarkable feature is the relationship between fiber size and fiber type in masseter muscle; fast-type fibers of masseter muscle have a smaller cross-sectional area than the slow-type fibers, whereas the reverse is true in the limb and trunk muscles. This characteristic facilitates an increase in the exchange of O2, improving the resistance to fatigue so that it is most advantageous for mastication.

It is clear that *both the macroscopic and microscopic characteristics of masticatory muscles (particularly the masseter) are special and notably different from limb and trunk muscles*. This is probably due to their refined motor control, which requires a continual regulation of force during mastication, and the complex coordination between the bolus side and the contralateral that these muscles must perform. In the light of these characteristics, we will go on to describe the coordinated activity of masticatory muscles during function.

3.8 Coordination of masticatory muscles during mastication

The characteristic of masticatory muscles that we must grasp in order to understand masticatory function is the coordination between sides, which is essential in diagnosing equilibrium or dyskinesia of mastication. The absolute EMG amplitude has little clinical significance as it is too variable to external factors to be considered as reliable data. On the contrary, coordination between the muscles of the bolus side and the contralateral represents the physiological aspect of the neuromuscular control of mastication. This is present and recurs constantly in any type of malocclusion, both before and after therapy. Muscle coordination, as opposed to EMG amplitude, is the subject of interest in our study; knowledge of this field is essential in understanding the positive clinical effects of physiological coordination or, vice versa, the negative effects of changes to the same.

3.8.1 Coordinated activity of masticatory muscles

Electrognathographic and EMG instruments allow us to acquire, simultaneously, mandibular kinetics and EMG activity readings of four of the eight masticatory muscles: right and left masseters, and right and left anterior temporalis muscles. This technological possibility, developed around 20 years ago, has proved of great importance in the understanding of chewing cycle alterations and the muscles involved.

However, there are eight masticatory muscles in total, which means that we are able to describe only half of the neuromuscular activity involved in mastication. Fortunately, the masseters and anterior temporalis muscles show a different significant role during chewing and are suitable for helping us to understand the muscular control. The system is extremely complex, and what we know today is surely just a small part. Further investigations are necessary to establish a deeper understanding of these phenomena, as our knowledge of motor control neurophysiology improves.

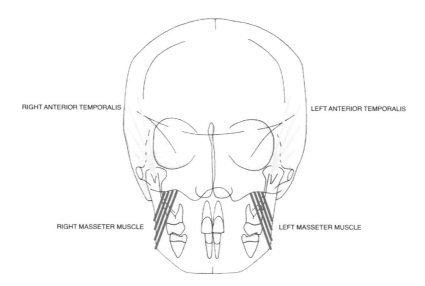

Figure 3.16   Schematic representation of anterior temporalis and masseter muscles.

3.8.2 Activation of the masseter and anterior temporalis muscles in patients with normal occlusion

In physiological conditions, the masseter and anterior temporalis muscles perform two very different roles (Figure 3.16). *The anterior temporalis muscles are responsible for controlling the position of the mandible in the space*, and we can view them as dynamic postural muscles rather than power muscles.

On the other hand, *masseter muscles are true power muscles* – highly coordinated, able to grind the bolus and to regulate their force thanks to precise neuromuscular control.

Given their different roles, it is logical that their coordination takes place differently between the two sides. The functional characteristics of each muscle are as follows (Figures 3.17, 3.18):

- Ipsilateral anterior temporalis muscle on the bolus side:
  - this activates prior to the contralateral side;
  - it achieves similar maximum activity levels to the contralateral side;
  - peak activity lasts for a very short period.
- Contralateral anterior temporalis muscle:
  - this activates after the ipsilateral side;
  - it achieves similar maximum activity levels to the ipsilateral side;
  - peak activity lasts for a very short period.
- Ipsilateral masseter muscle on the bolus side:
  - this achieves twice the activity of the contralateral side;
  - activity increases gradually until a defined peak is reached;
  - its activity decreases quickly.
- Contralateral masseter muscle:
  - this activates before the ipsilateral side;
  - it achieves significantly lower electrical activity than the ipsilateral side;
  - its activity decreases slowly.

3.8.2.1 *The anterior temporalis*

It appears clear that the anterior temporalis muscles activate in a similar and symmetric way between the two sides, and that the difference between the sides resides in the *time period* of activation when comparing the bolus side with the contralateral side.

This is important in controlling the position of the mandible in space whilst masseter force is expressed. Unfortunately, the anterior temporalis muscle may be engaged in crosstalk with the masseter, and this can produce inaccurate readings of EMG values.

3.8.2.2. *The masseter*

The masseter is an extremely complex and refined muscle, characterized by asymmetric activity during the single chewing cycle, and the same muscle may assume different roles according to whether it is on the bolus or on the contralateral side. In fact, *the masseter of the bolus side is the real power muscle*, responsible for bolus grinding, whilst *the contralateral masseter performs a regulatory role of the mandibular position in the space*, being the first to activate, and counterbalancing the prevailing masseter action on the bolus side. A morphological difference in EMG activity can also be seen. In fact, the contralateral masseter does not display activity with peaks, like the bolus side, but exhibits instead a plateau-type performance characterized by slowly decreasing activity. This morphological difference of the EMG tracing is related to the function, with peak activity being necessary in order to generate power for grinding, whereas plateau-type activity is suitable for postural control of the mandible in the space.

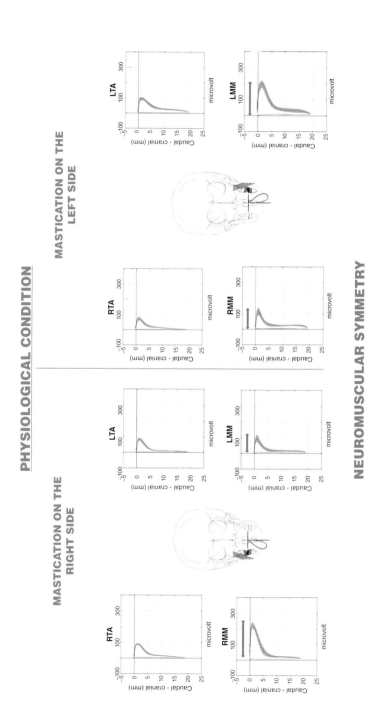

Figure 3.17 Electromyography tracings of anterior temporalis and masseter during physiologic alternate chewing showing the neuromuscular balance between sides. RTA: right anterior temporalis, LTA: left anterior temporalis, RMM: right masseter muscle; LMM: left masseter muscle. Green tracings: opening; red tracings: closing.

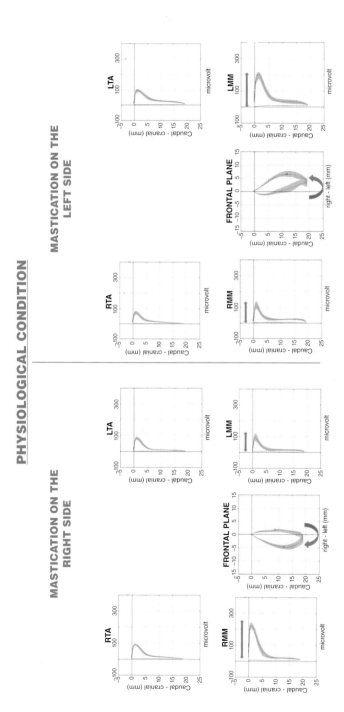

Figure 3.18 The chewing pattern simultaneously recorded with the electromyography of both sides of the anterior temporalis and masseter muscles during physiologic alternate chewing showing the neuromuscular balance between sides. RTA: right anterior temporalis; LTA: left anterior temporalis; RMM: right masseter muscle; LMM: left masseter muscle. Green tracings: opening; red tracings: closing.

Iacoboni M. (2008) *I neuroni a specchio. Come capiamo ciò che fanno gli altri*. Bollati Boringhieri Editore, Turin.

Igarashi Y, Aita M, Suzuki A, *et al.* (2007) Involvement of GDNF and its receptors in the maturation of the periodontal Ruffini endings. *Neurosci Lett* 412, 222–226.

Ishida T, Yabushita T, Ono T. (2013) Functional reversibility of temporomandibular joint mechanoreceptors. *Arch Oral Biol* 58(9), 1078–1083.

Ishii N, Soma K, Toda K. (2002) Response properties of periodontal mechanoreceptors in rats, in vitro. *Brain Res Bull* 58(4), 357–361.

Johnsen SE, Trulsson M. (2003) Receptive field properties of human periodontal afferents responding to loading of premolar and molar teeth. *J Neurophysiol* 89(3), 1478–1487.

Johnston CA, Tyler C, Stansberry SA, *et al.* (2012) Brief report: gum chewing affects standardized math scores in adolescents. *J Adolesc* 35(2), 455–459.

Kandel ER, Schwartz JH, Jessel TM, *et al.* (eds) (2012) *Principles of neural science*, 5th edn. McGraw-Hill, New York.

Kawahata M, Ono Y, Ohno A, *et al.* (2014) Loss of molars early in life develops behavioral lateralization and impairs hippocampus-dependent recognition memory. *BMC Neurosci* 15, 4.

Kawanishi K, Koshino H, Toyoshita Y, *et al.* (2010) Effect of mastication on functional recoveries after permanent middle cerebral artery occlusion in rats. *J Stroke Cerebrovasc Dis* 19(5), 398–403.

Kiliaridis S, Engström C, Thilander B. (1985) The relationship between masticatory function and craniofacial morphology. I. A cephalometric longitudinal analysis in the growing rat fed a soft diet. *Eur J Orthod* 7(4), 273–283.

Kimura Y, Ogawa H, Yoshihara A, *et al.* (2013) Evaluation of chewing ability and its relationship with activities of daily living, depression, cognitive status and food intake in the community-dwelling elderly. *Geriatr Gerontol Int* 13(3), 718–725.

Korfage JA, Koolstra JH, Langenbach GE, van Eijden TM. (2005) Fiber-type composition of the human jaw muscles – (part 1) origin and functional significance of fiber-type diversity. *J Dent Res* 84(9), 774–783.

Komuro A, Masuda Y, Iwata K, *et al.* (2001) Influence of food thickness and hardness on possible feed-forward control of the masseteric muscle activity in the anesthetized rabbit. *Neurosci Res* 39(1), 21–29.

Lexomboon D, Trulsson M, Wardh I, Parker MG. (2012) Chewing ability and tooth loss: association with cognitive impairment in an elderly population study. *J Am Geriatr Soc* 60(10), 1951–1956.

Linden RW, Scott BJ. (1989) Distribution of mesencephalic nucleus and trigeminal ganglion mechanoreceptors in the periodontal ligament of the cat. *J Physiol* 410, 35–44.

Lund JP, Kolta A. (2006) Generation of the central masticatory pattern and its modification by sensory feedback. *Dysphagia* 21(3), 167–174.

Lund JP, Scott G, Kolta A, Westeberg GR. (1999) Role of cortical inputs and brainstem interneuron, populations in patterning mastication. In: *Neurobiology of mastication. From molecular to system approach* (eds Y Nakamura, GJ Sessle). Elsevier, Tokyo, pp. 504–514.

Maeda T, Ochi K, Nakakuma-Ohshima K, *et al.* (1999) The Ruffini ending as the primary mechanoreceptor in the periodontal ligament: its morphology, cytochemical features, regeneration, and development. *Crit Rev Oral Biol Med* 10(3), 307–327.

Maruyama Y, Harada F, Jabbar S, *et al.* (2005) Neurotrophin-4/5-depletion induces a delay in maturation of the periodontal Ruffini endings in mice. *Arch Histol Cytol* 68, 267–288.

Masood M, Masood Y, Newton T. (2014) Cross-bite and oral health related quality of life in young people. *J Dent* 42(3), 249–255.

Masuda Y, Kato T, Hidaka O, *et al.* (2001) Neuronal activity in the putamen and the globus pallidus of rabbit during mastication. *Neurosci Res* 39(1), 11–19.

Merletti R (ed.). (1999) *SENIAM – raccomandazioni europee per l' elettromiografia di superficie*. CLUT, Turin.

Merletti R (ed.). (2000) *Elementi di elettromiografia di superficie*. CLUT, Turin.

Merlo A, Campanini I. (2010) Technical aspects of surface electromyography for clinicians. *Open Rehabil J* 3, 98–109.

Merlo A, Farina D, Merletti R (2003) A fast and reliable technique for muscle activity detection from surface EMG signals. *IEEE Trans Biomed Eng* 50(3), 316–323.

Mioche L, Peyron MA. (1995) Bite force displaced during assessment of hardness in various texture contexts. *Arch Oral Biol* 40(5), 415–423.

Mioche L, Bourdiol P, Martin JF, Noel Y. (1999) Variations in human masseter and temporalis muscle activity related to food texture during free and side imposed mastication. *Arch Oral Biol* 44(12), 1005–1012.

Miyawaki S, Ohkochi N, Kawakami T, Sugimura M. (2001) Changes in masticatory muscle activity according to food size in experimental human mastication. *J Oral Rehabil* 28(8), 778–784.

Moller E. (1966) The chewing apparatus. An electromyographic study of the action of the muscles of mastication and its correlation to facial morphology. *Acta Physiol Scand* 69(Suppl 280), 1–229.

Moller E. (1969) Clinical electromyography in dentistry. *Int Dent J* 19(2), 250–266.

Moller E. (1974) Action of the muscles of mastication. *Front Oral Physiol* 1(0):121–158.

Morimoto T, Inoue T, Nakamura T, Kawamura Y. (1984) Frequency-dependent modulation of rhythmic human jaw movements. *J Dent Res* 63(11), 1310–1314.

Morquette P, Lavoie R, Fhima MD, *et al.* (2012) Generation of the masticatory central pattern and its modulation by sensory feedback. *Prog Neurobiol* 96(3), 340–355.

Moss ML. (1968) A theoretical analysis of the functional matrix. *Acta Biotheor* 18(1), 195–202.

Naeije M, Hofman N. (2003) Biomechanics of the human temporomandibular joint during chewing. *J Dent Res* 82(7), 528–531.

Nagata K, Itoh S, Tsuboi A, *et al.* (2008) Response properties of periodontal mechanosensitive neurons in the trigeminal ganglion of rabbit and neuronal activities during grinding-like jaw movement induced by cortical stimulation. *Arch Oral Biol* 53(12), 1138–1148.

Nakakura-Ohshima K, Maeda T, Ohshima H, *et al.* (1995) Postnatal development of periodontal Ruffini endings in rat incisors: an immunoelectron microscopic study using protein gene product 9.5 (PGP 9.5) antibody. *J Comp Neurol* 362(4), 551–564.

Narita N, Kamiya K, Yamamura K, *et al.* (2009) Chewing-related prefrontal cortex activation while wearing partial denture prosthesis: pilot study. *J Prosthodont Res* 53(3), 126–135.

Neff P. (1999) *Occlusion and function.* Georgetown University School of Dentistry, Washington, DC. http://peterneffdds.com/blog, http://www.amazon.com/TMJ-occlusion-function-Peter-Neff/dp/B0006RE5SK (accessed October 2, 2015).

Nishino H, Hattori S, Muramoto K, Ono T. (1991) Basal ganglia neural activity during operant feeding behavior in the monkey: relation to sensory integration and motor execution. *Brain Res Bull* 27(3–4), 463–468.

Ochi K, Wakisaka S, Youn SH, *et al.* (1997) Calretinin-like immunoreactivity in the Ruffini endings, slowly adapting mechanoreceptors, of the periodontal ligament of the rat incisor. *Brain Res* 769(1), 183–187.

Ohishi M, Harada F, Rahman F, *et al.* (2009) GDNF expression in terminal Schwann cells associated with the periodontal Ruffini endings of the rat incisors during nerve regeneration. *Anat Rec (Hoboken)* 292(8), 1185–1191.

Ono Y, Yamamoto T, Kubo KY, Onozuka M. (2010) Occlusion and brain function: mastication as a prevention of cognitive dysfunction. *J Oral Rehabil* 37(8), 624–640.

Onyper SV, Carr TL, Farrar JS, Floyd BR. (2011) Cognitive advantages of chewing gum. Now you see them, now you don't. *Appetite* 57(2), 321–328.

Piancino MG, Bracco P, Vallelonga T, *et al.* (2008) Effect of bolus hardness on the chewing pattern and activation of masticatory muscles in subjects with normal dental occlusion. *J Electromyogr Kinesiol* 18(6), 931–937.

Purves D, Augustine GJ, Fitzpatrick D, *et al.* (2009) *Neuroscienze* (trans RLucchi, APoli). Zanichelli, Bologna.

Roatta S, Windhorst U, Ljubisavljevic M, *et al.* (2002) Sympathetic modulation of muscle spindle afferent sensitivity to stretch in rabbit jaw closing muscles. *J Physiol* 540(Pt 1), 237–248.

Roatta S, Windhorst U, Djupsjöbacka M, *et al.* (2005) Effects of sympathetic stimulation on the rhythmical jaw movements produced by electrical stimulation of the cortical masticatory areas of rabbits. *Exp Brain Res* 162(1), 14–22.

Rizzolatti G, Craighero L. (2004) The mirror-neuron system. *Annu Rev Neurosci* 27, 169–192.

Rizzolatti G, Sinigaglia C. (2010) The functional role of the parieto-frontal mirror circuit: interpretations and misinterpretations. *Nat Rev Neurosci* 11(4), 264–274.

Rizzolatti G, Fadiga L, Gallese V, Fogassi L. (1996) Premotor cortex and the recognition of motor actions. *Brain Res Cogn Brain Res* 3(2), 131–141.

Shi L, Atsumi Y, Kodama Y, *et al.* (2006) Requirement of proper occlusal force for morphological maturation of neural components of periodontal Ruffini endings of the rat incisor. *Arch Oral Biol* 51(8), 681–688.

Shoi K, Fueki K, Usui N, *et al.* (2014) Influence of posterior dental arch length on brain activity during chewing in patients with mandibular distal extension removable partial dentures. *J Oral Rehabil* 41(7), 486–495.

Smith A. (2010) Effects of chewing gum on cognitive function, mood and physiology in stressed and non-stressed volunteers. *Nutr Neurosci* 13(1), 7–16.

Sodeyama T, Maeda T, Takano Y, Hara K. (1996) Responses of periodontal nerve terminals to experimentally induced occlusal trauma in rat molars: an immunohistochemical study using PGP 9.5 antibody. *J Period Res* 31(4), 235–248.

Tabata T, Hayashi H. (1994) Physiological properties of periodontal mechanosensitive neurones in the trigeminal (Gasserian) ganglion of the rat. *Arch Oral Biol* 39(5), 379–385.

Tabata T, Yamaki A, Takahashi Y, Hayashi H. (2002) Physiological properties of periodontal mechanosensitive neurones in the posteromedial ventral nucleus of rat thalamus. *Arch Oral Biol* 47(9), 689–694.

Tabata T, Takahashi Y, Hayashi H. (2006) Physiological properties of molar-mechanosensitive periodontal neurons in the trigeminal ganglion of the rat. *Arch Oral Biol* 51(9), 729–735.

Takada T, Miyamoto T. (2004) A fronto-parietal network for chewing of gum: a study on human subjects with functional magnetic resonance imaging. *Neurosci Lett* 360(3), 137–140.

Teixeira FB, Pereira Fernandes LdeM, Noronha PA, *et al.* (2014) Masticatory deficiency as a risk factor for cognitive dysfunction. *Int J Med Sci* 11(2), 209–214.

Thilander B. (1995) Basic mechanisms in craniofacial growth. *Acta Odont Scand* 53(3), 144–151.

Thilander B, Carlsson GE, Ingerval B. (1976) Postnatal Development of the human temporomandibular joint. I. A histological study. *Acta Odont Scand* 34, 117–126.

Toda T, Taoka M. (2001) The complexity of receptive fields of periodontal mechanoreceptive neurons in the postcentral area 2 of conscious macaque monkey brains. *Arch Oral Biol* 46(11), 1079–1084.

Trulsson M, Essick GK. (2010) Sensations evoked by microstimulation of single mechanoreceptive afferents innervating the human face and mouth. *J Neurophysiol* 103(4), 1741–1747.

Trulsson M, Francis ST, Bowtell R, McGlone F. (2010) Brain activations in response to vibrotactile tooth stimulation: a psychophysical and fMRI study. *J Neurophysiol* 104(4), 2257–2265.

Tsuboi A, Takafuji Y, Itoh S, *et al.* (2009) Response properties of trigeminal ganglion mechanosensitive neurons innervating the temporomandibular joint of the rabbit. *Exp Brain Res* 199(2), 107–116.

Umemura T, Yasuda K, Ishihama K, *et al.* (2010) A comparison of the postnatal development of muscle-spindle and periodontal-ligament neurons in the mesencephalic trigeminal nucleus of the rat. *Neurosci Lett* 473, 155–157.

Weijenberg RA, Scherder EJ, Lobbezoo F. (2011) Mastication for the mind – the relationship between mastication and cognition in ageing and dementia. *Neurosci Biobehav Rev* 35(3), 483–497.

Woda A. (1984) *Fisiologia del sistema stomatognatico*. Elsevier–Masson, Milan.

Yu H, Chen X, Liu J, Zhou X. (2013) Gum chewing inhibits the sensory processing and the propagation of stress-related information in a brain network. *PLoS ONE* 8(4), e57111.

Chapter 4

Alterations to Masticatory Function in Unilateral Crossbites

Contents

Understanding Masticatory Function in Unilateral Crossbites, First Edition. Maria Grazia Piancino and Stephanos Kyrkanides.
© 2016 John Wiley & Sons, Inc. Published 2016 by John Wiley & Sons, Inc.

4.1 Introduction

The study of masticatory disorders must not overlook the experience and clinical skill of researchers, who, in this field, cannot rely exclusively on technology and mathematics. Obviously, a statistic-based result of data is a fundamental reference point in accurately identifying a phenomenon, but the research project must evolve around clinical significance and not simply statistical figures (Figure 4.1). The risk of such a solely statistical approach in this field may lead to the diffusion of results that that are ambiguous from a clinical point of view. Thus, a clinical-significance approach was adopted in the Orthognathodontic Faculty of the University of Turin–Italy, where malocclusions and their functional consequences were diagnosed and studied daily. This activity has led to the observation of masticatory function during the early stages of child development – before, after, and during treatment.

The use of the instruments explained in chapter 1 allowed us, from the very start, to study mandibular movement alongside electromyographic (EMG) activity of the masseter and anterior temporalis muscles. This was very important to relate the two issues of masticatory pattern and

FROM PHYSIOLOGY TO ALTERATION OF THE MASTICATORY SYSTEM

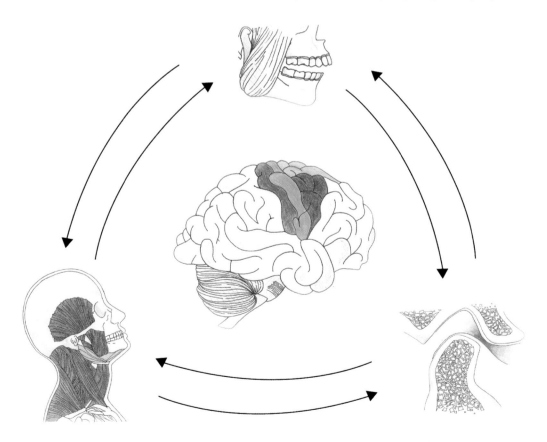

Figure 4.1   The masticatory system. *Source for the muscles:* Neff (1999). *Source for the brain:* Purves *et al.* (2000). Reproduced with the permission of Sinauer Associates.

neuromuscular activation for a better understanding of masticatory function. The results were achieved on the basis of clinical experience, and statistically confirmed for increased significance.

There are many examples of malocclusions that modify the chewing cycle, but for the purposes of simplicity and clarity in such a complex topic as mastication, this book will limit itself to one phenomenon in two variations: *unilateral posterior and anterior crossbite.*

These malocclusions, which are each very different even though they belong to the same chapter, influence the chewing cycle in a different and repeatable way. Conversely, modifications to the chewing cycle represent the etiopathogenesis of signs and symptoms that a mere study of the malposition of teeth cannot reveal. Thus, *the real aim of orthognathodontic therapy*, especially during developmental stages, is *to rebalance all the elements of the stomatognathic system* in order to restore healthy function and growth. This diagnostic and therapeutic approach is still relatively rare in the orthognathodontic field for a number of reasons, but principally due to the invasive role wrongly attributed to the technical aspects related to equipment. The study and comprehension of mastication can bring about a physiological evolution, which is the way to achieve a "healthy stomatognathic system."

4.2 Crossbite=neuromuscular syndrome (Figure 4.2)

Unilateral crossbite and its effects on chewing pattern is an ideal way to understand masticatory function, but to do so we need to understand its etiopathogenetic and clinical features. *Crossbite* is a malocclusion that is first diagnosed via the teeth, although the effects and symptoms related to dental malposition represent just a small part of the impact of crossbite. In fact, crossbite affects mastication, neuromuscular coordination, neural motor memory, the inner skeletal structure, the TMJ, and all of the stomatognathic system with its related structures (Moller and Troelstrup, 1975; Bracco *et al.*, 2002). It is characterized by two special features: the type of asymmetry and the early age of onset.

Asymmetry (dental, skeletal and/or positional) is one of the unique and particular features of crossbite, along with its consequential functional effects: it may originate from a skeletal or dental malrelationship, or both, and may lead to a mandibular displacement. The second feature is *the early age at which it may emerge*, during eruption of the primary dentition, and it can involve the permanent dentition at a later stage of development. It has an influence on masticatory function and the effects will worsen over time and are irreversible once the growth stage is complete.

Thus, it is clear that the definition of crossbite as a "malocclusion" is extremely restrictive and that it would be more accurate and useful from a diagnostic point of view to define crossbite as a "neuromuscular syndrome." This is its real defining characteristic, and the approach we wish to take in developing a suitable therapy for functional correction and "cure" of the patient's stomatognathic system. Teeth are the means via which we can currently achieve this goal. However, when teeth become the be-all and end-all of this issue, instead of merely a means, then any type of reasoning based on function may become difficult to understand. Modern-day technology offers us many orthodontic devices capable of correcting dental misalignment caused by crossbite in relatively simple procedures, but functional repair is still far from being a routine affair. We may say that what is required today in the orthodontic field is not so much technological innovation as the pursuit and sharing of physiological and pathological knowledge regarding crossbite function and its consequences.

To understand modifications to mastication, we need, first, to *view and analyze the biological and clinical features of crossbite as an asymmetric and worsening* "neuromuscular syndrome." Therefore, we will first give the definition, etiology, and dental/skeletal function classifications of crossbite

PATHOLOGY OF MASTICATION

CROSSBITE = NEUROMUSCULAR SYNDROME

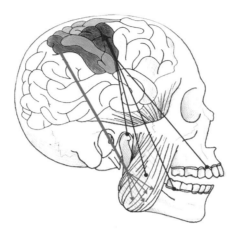

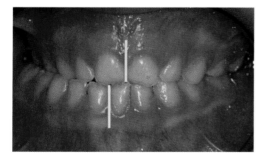 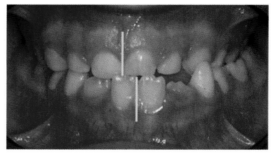

It is of clinical relevance, for successful orthodontic treatment, to consider not only the repositioning of teeth within the dental arches, but also, and above all, the effects of therapy on function.

Figure 4.2   Right and left unilateral posterior crossbite malocclusions: a neuromuscular syndrome.

in general terms as well as those of unilateral crossbite in particular, along with clinical consequences. This is followed by a detailed description of alterations to mastication (subdivided into objectives), thus avoiding the reduction of masticatory study to a futile mathematical–statistical exercise, in an attempt to comprehend the clinical importance of masticatory function.

4.2.1 Definition

Crossbite is described as a serious asymmetric and worsening malocclusion.

Bjork *et al.* (1964) defined crossbite as a malocclusion that may affect *"the canine, premolar and molar region*, characterized by the buccal cusps of the maxillary teeth occluding lingual to the buccal cusps of the corresponding mandibular teeth." The advantage of this "archaic" but clinically significant definition is that it subdivides the teeth regions according to different functions.

More recently, in 2002, the *Glossary of Orthodontic Terms* describes crossbite as an anomalous relationship of one or more teeth with one or more elements of the opposite dental arch, in the buccal–lingual or labial–lingual direction adding that a crossbite may be either *dental or skeletal* in origin (Daskalogiannakis, 2002). This "modern" definition recognizes that the skeletal role plays an integral part in the malocclusion. In the light of current knowledge, we can add that crossbite is connected *to worsening structural and functional asymmetry*.

4.2.2 Prevalence

The prevalence of crossbite is reported in the literature as being between 8 and 22% (Harrison and Ashby, 2003). According to a study carried out at the Dental School of the University of Turin–Italy (Piancino *et al.*, 2006a) on 5300 patients aged between 6 and 16 years old (Figures 4.3 and 4.4), with malocclusions requiring orthodontic treatment, crossbite was diagnosed in 19% of the cases.

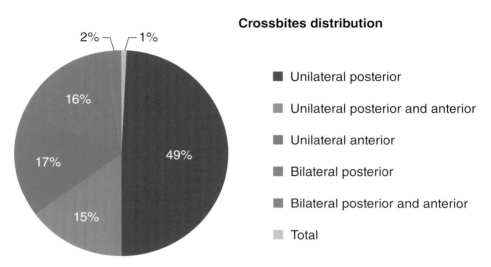

Crossbites distribution

- ■ Unilateral posterior
- ■ Unilateral posterior and anterior
- ■ Unilateral anterior
- ■ Bilateral posterior
- ■ Bilateral posterior and anterior
- ■ Total

Figure 4.3 Distribution of crossbites in Italian orthodontic population.

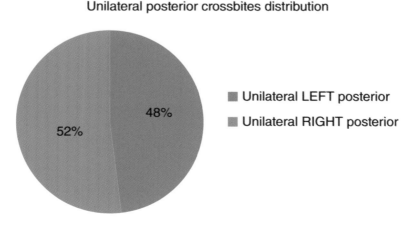

Unilateral posterior crossbites distribution

- ■ Unilateral LEFT posterior
- ■ Unilateral RIGHT posterior

Figure 4.4 Distribution of right and left unilateral posterior crossbites in Italian orthodontic population *Source:* Piancino *et al.* (2006a). Reproduced with permission from Oxford University Press.

Around half of these displayed unilateral posterior crossbite (51% on the right-hand side and 49% on the left). From the total number of crossbite cases, 49% displayed unilateral posterior crossbite, 16% bilateral posterior; 17% anterior only, 15% unilateral anterior and posterior crossbite, 2% bilateral anterior and posterior, and 1% total. Some studies (da Silva Filho *et al.*, 2007) on the prevalence of unilateral crossbite, carried out on children aged between 3 and 6 years old, revealed that deciduous dentition displayed crossbite condition in 20% of cases, 11% of which regarded unilateral posterior crossbite. These results can be matched with those in the literature on children aged 6–16 years old with deciduous and permanent dentition. However, the results are decidedly different regarding bilateral posterior crossbite; in this case, 1.19% was recorded for deciduous dentition as opposed to the 16% recorded for mixed deciduous and permanent dentition. Furthermore, in children with deciduous dentition, the study reveals the presence of functional positional crossbite in 91% of cases (3–6 years of age) as opposed to the 67% reported in the literature for patients aged between 7 and 12 years old with mixed dentition (Pinto *et al.*, 2001).

The clinical significance of these results is that in toddlers and very young children, *the most common crossbite condition is unilateral posterior crossbite*, which is related to worsening structural and functional dissymmetry. Thus, the sooner this abnormality is diagnosed and corrected, the sooner correct functioning and growth will be restored. The later the correction occurs, the more likely it is that basal asymmetry will evolve, with irreversible effects for function.

In later childhood, the cases of bilateral crossbite become more common; this is a malocclusion caused, above all, by a serious incongruity in the maxillary skeletal development on the transversal plane.

4.2.3 Etiology

Many causes may lie behind this type of malocclusion. Apart from *hereditary factors*, which are often the basis of crossbites characterized by the simultaneous presence of maxillary hypoplasia and mandibular prognathism, attention must be paid to *functional changes* such as oral respiration, *abnormal patterns of deglutition* (Figure 4.5) and *bad habits* such as thumb-sucking (Figure 4.6) or the excessive use of dummies and baby bottles. Other causes include congenital alterations such as *labial palatal clefts, dystrophic alterations, metabolism disorders, infections or trauma* – in other words, all pathologies which slow down or alter the growth of the upper maxillary, thus causing the hypoplasia.

Environmental factors also play a part; for example, the *agenesis or premature extraction of one or more teeth*, which decreases the functional matrix of the upper maxillary during childhood development.

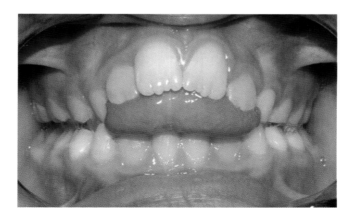

Figure 4.5 Tongue thrusting.

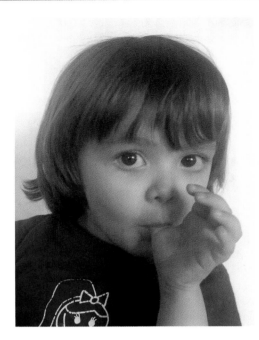

Figure 4.6 Thumb-sucking.

As we will explain later, the importance of masticatory function and modified chewing patterns in this malocclusion is clear. So far, we are unable to determine whether (and to what extent) the motor pattern of mastication may influence the emergence of crossbite in the early stages of deciduous dentition. Or, more precisely, we know that, usually, in cases of posterior crossbite, mastication is altered and establishes an anomalous and asymmetric pattern that is highly resistant to change; but we still do not know whether there might be cases in which this atypical pattern is neurologically inherited as such, and whether it influences the occlusion (thus contributing to the emergence of a crossbite condition). We hope that research will be able to answer this question one day, thus allowing the development of new preventive therapies.

4.2.4 Functional classification

Crossbite is characterized by *an inverse relationship (on the frontal and/or sagittal plane)* of one or more teeth in which the buccal cusps and/or upper incisal margins occlude palatally with the buccal cusps and/or lower incisal margins, *on either one or both sides of the dental arches.* It is, then, an extremely complex and varying malocclusion, which may involve different types and numbers of teeth.

For this reason, a classification is necessary. The classification of a malocclusion must be viewed, by both professionals and students, as a type of navigational compass: far from being a static and meaningless definition, the categorization of various types of crossbite according to dynamic and functional characteristics allows us to move in the right diagnostic and/or therapeutic direction. Furthermore, it helps create a shared scientific terminology.

The task of classifying crossbite conditions is complex because, as stated earlier, it involves teeth, cranial structures, and neuromuscular and articular function. This is why dental classification, although important, is not sufficient per se and must be combined with functional and

THE FUNCTIONAL ROLE OF TEETH

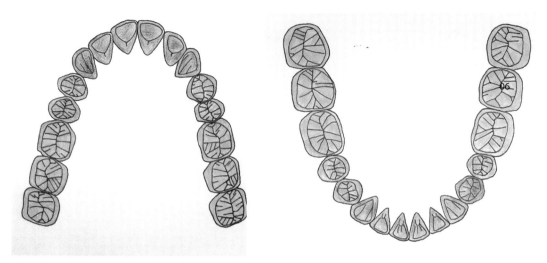

Figure 4.7 Anterior and posterior functional region of the occlusion. The diagram in two colours demonstrates the dual role of premolars, which provide support as well as dynamic control. *Source:* Slavicek (2002). Reproduced with permission from R. Slavicek.

basal classification if a correct diagnosis is to be made. However, *dental classification* is a good starting point in the process for two reasons:

1. A crossbite condition may affect any number and any type of teeth.
2. Depending on the region of the malocclusion, the effects on function may differ.

Thus, it is clear that a universal classification system and common terminology are necessary. To understand functional classification of crossbite, we need to remember that the functional role of teeth in humans differs according to the region in question. The dental arches may be divided into two main areas, anterior and posterior, with the functional roles of these regions being very different (Slavicek, 2002) (Figure 4.7).

The anterior contact region (from upper and lower canine to canine) features teeth that, in terms of anatomic morphology, do not make intercuspid contact but do make contact between the upper and lower arch to perform a role of *"sensory control" and guidance of the mandible in space, as well as protecting the diatoric contacts thanks to the laterotrusive and protrusive gliding areas*. The guide function takes place in the frontal area – in fact, the majority of contacts during activity are to be found in the functional lingual surface of the upper incisors. The anterior region may be viewed as a true sensory organ.

The posterior region (upper and lower molars), on the other hand, features teeth that make intercuspid contact with each other, thus helping support occlusion during functional movements and grinding of the bolus during mastication. It is the region entrusted with mastication.

The middle contact area (upper and lower premolars) features teeth that make intercuspid contact as well as contributing to laterotrusive control. In this sense they differ from molars, which provide a primary role in support and mastication – the premolars provide an important intermediary stage between the anterior control area and the posterior area of support and grinding.

UNILATERAL CROSSBITE = ASYMMETRIC NEUROMUSCULAR SYNDROME

Posterior crossbite multiple teeth

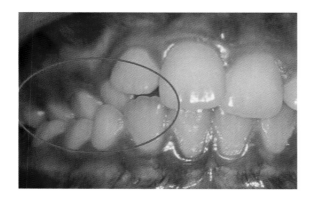
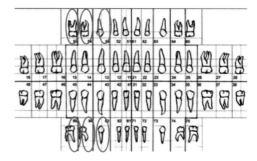

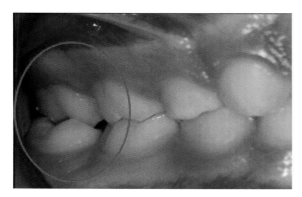
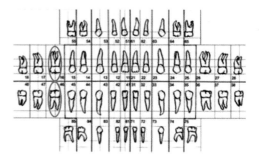

Posterior crossbite one tooth

Figure 4.8 Unilateral posterior crossbite involving multiple teeth (*top*) and one tooth (*bottom*).

The functional division of the upper dental arch is similar to that of the lower anterior area (incisor and canine), the posterior area (molar), and intermediary area (premolar), apart from the lower first premolar, which is functionally included in the laterotrusive control. This corresponds to the gnathological concept of organic occlusion – the contrast between the different functional fields of the individual dental groups supplies a mutual protection function in the different dental arches (Slavicek, 2002). On the basis of this knowledge, it is easy to see that the alteration of masticatory function correlates to the functional region involved by the malocclusion.

Correct diagnosis of crossbite requires a dental classification based on the concepts of organic occlusion, as outlined above (Figures 4.8 and 4.9). Based on these gnathological concepts, tables for dental classification of crossbite have been produced. These subdivide the malocclusion into anterior, middle, and posterior regions, but it must be added that crossbite may affect just one hemiarch or both arches bilaterally, with significant different functional effects and impact on functional structural development. Therefore, it is necessary to first subdivide the crossbite conditions into unilateral or bilateral categories.

UNILATERAL CROSSBITE = ASYMMETRIC NEUROMUSCULAR SYNDROME

Anterior crossbite

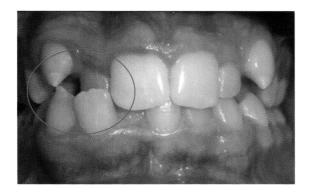
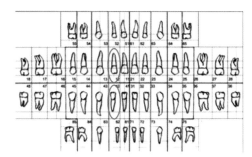

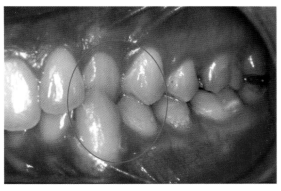
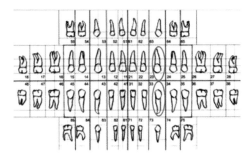

Canine crossbite

Figure 4.9   Unilateral anterior (*top*) and canine (*bottom*) crossbite.

This chapter will look solely at unilateral crossbites, as the bilateral condition is an extremely complex malocclusion requiring in-depth and careful analysis from functional, diagnostic, and therapeutic viewpoints.

4.3 Unilateral posterior crossbite

4.3.1 Definition

Unilateral posterior crossbite may be defined as a malocclusion where one or more posterior maxillary teeth have a more palatal or lingual position than the corresponding antagonist mandibular tooth (or teeth), on one side only of the dental arch only.

As explained previously, *precise dental and basal classification* is of aid in diagnosing and treating unilateral posterior crossbite. For example, median line deviation (often present in this condition) may be caused by mandibular displacement, dental malposition, basal asymmetry, or these factors together. Differential diagnosis, as far as possible, is important to identify the most suitable treatment, and the correct dental/basal classification helps in selecting the best focused personalized treatments.

4.3.2 Dental classification

As already described, unilateral posterior crossbite concerns the premolar and molar regions on one side only of the dental arch.

It may concern one or more teeth, thus constituting two subgroups:

• unilateral posterior crossbite of a single tooth;
• unilateral posterior crossbite of multiple teeth.

Dental classification of crossbite regards just one aspect of the malocclusion and thus needs to be supported by basal classification also. However, before looking at skeletal aspects, we would like to point out that teeth (with their periodontal mechanoreceptors and rigid structure) determine all the functional processes of mastication. *Occlusal asymmetry* in unilateral posterior crossbite is very clear and involves the dental cusps, which are participatory in masticatory function. In light of this fact, we now introduce the basal classification, which is closely linked to the important function of mastication.

4.3.3 Basal classification

As always in orthognathodontics, dental classification must be used in conjunction with basal classification.

Crossbite is a unique malocclusion that is complex, worsening, and characterized by the fact that, starting with the teeth, *it involves all the elements of the stomatognathic system in the three spatial dimensions*, together with all its functions. The most evident feature of this malocclusion is asymmetry (basal and functional), which causes the ingravescence and irreversibility of the side effects once growth has ended. The asymmetry of unilateral posterior crossbite is extremely complex and regards all three spatial planes, which must be evaluated for a comprehensive diagnosis. The asymmetry of unilateral posterior crossbite can originate from altered dental (and/or skeletal) relations and may lead to displacement or malposition of the mandible. Thus, it may display both static and dynamic features; this is a special aspect of the asymmetry of this malocclusion.

In contrast with dental classification, basal classification does not identify well-defined and independent groups but involves the *dominance of one skeletal feature over another*. In the early stages of development, the most common condition is positional or functional unilateral posterior crossbite that evolves gradually in stages to become dento-alveolar crossbite and, eventually, dento-alveolar–basal crossbite. This classification is a guide to understand the evolution of the malocclusion, but it is clear that each case is a case in itself that may show different timing, different environmental or genetic influence, and, at the end, a different evolution.

Thus, the basal classification of unilateral posterior crossbite is:

1. positional or functional;
2. dento-alveolar;
3. dento-alveolar-basal.

4.3.3.1 *Positional or functional crossbite* (Figure 4.10)

This type of crossbite is very particular, widespread, and unique within its genre. Thus, it is essential to diagnose it as quickly and accurately as possible in order to proceed with the appropriate treatment. Usually, *the condition emerges during early infancy (between 2 and 5 years of age) and results in a deflected dental contact that causes an asymmetric lateral shift of the mandible.* When the first contact position is in place (i.e., when the mandible is in a centered position), cuspid-to-cuspid dental contacts are established between the upper and lower teeth. The *inputs generated by the dental mechanoreceptors* are received and elaborated by the central nervous system, activating masticatory muscles and deviating the mandible as it searches for a position of maximum intercuspation that is stable and

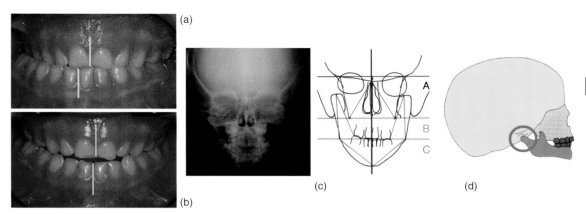

Figure 4.10 Positional or functional crossbite: occlusion in maximum intercuspation (a) and in centered position (b). Postero-anterior cephalometry (c: frontal plane): observe that in centered position the asymmetries, even if they are present, are not detectable. Representation of the deciduous stage of development (d: sagittal plane): the TMJ and the mandibular bone are clearly immature. *Source:* The representation of the deciduous stage has been redrawn from Slavicek (2002). Reproduced with permission from R. Slavicek.

necessary for any type of function, avoiding those input signals. Dental stability and the avoidance of cusp-to-cusp contacts are essential in allowing the vital functions of the stomatognathic system (i.e., deglutition and mastication) to be carried out. In other words, the system *"compensates"* (adapts in a pathological way see "Terminology") for the occlusal error of crossbite, trying to obtain the best function. However, it is not able to correct the defect, and the resulting biological consequences over time are unfortunately serious. In fact, owing to the early age at which this malocclusion occurs, *all developing structures will unbalance the mandibular shift and functional asymmetry*.

The most frequent cause of this type of crossbite is undoubtedly *hypoplasia of the upper maxilla* (the origins of which should be analyzed), and this is the diagnosis to take into account when tackling crossbite. Obviously, treatment should be planned accordingly. The persistent displacement of the mandible and the inversion of the relationship between dental cusps and asymmetric functional compensation causes a growing child to suffer disharmonious development.

This is the developmental stage during which a child learns all the motor skills, such as walking, climbing, chewing, deeply influencing and adapting the inherited automatism of the motor control of the central nervous system to the peripheral inputs. As Slavicek (2002) stated, oral functions (language, mastication, and deglutition) are "formative," and any dysfunction of these may influence the development of the masticatory system, disturbing its morphological and functional growth. It can be deduced then that "the assumption that maxillary abnormalities are genetically conditioned is not always accurate, because in the period of deciduous dental growth the system develops the best possible teeth for optimal functioning. And so, functional asymmetry may lead to morphological asymmetry. It would be a huge mistake to allow such asymmetries to develop," but early therapies must be physiological, avoiding traumatism.

One of the structures most involved is certainly the TMJ, because it is practically unformed at the time of birth. This anatomical feature has the functional purpose of allowing mandibular movements on the sagittal plane during breastfeeding. Thus, almost all temporomandibular and mandibular growth and development takes place post-birth. As histological studies have shown (Thilander *et al.*, 1976; Enlow, 1986; Thilander, 1995), *the growth of the TMJ is of adaptive type*; the adaptation of the joint is related to many factors: occlusion, cranial structure, muscles, functions, and so on. This means that such an asymmetric malocclusion, as well as inflammatory systemic diseases, causes considerable effects on growing structures, from both static and dynamic points of view (Piancino *et al.*, 2015a).

We will see how early orthodontic intervention in such cases may rebalance the function of the stomatognathic system and the growth of its structures, on condition that the therapeutic treatment be appropriate and avoids any type of dental trauma. Of course, it is true that early treatment is a chance, but the type of therapy is even more important.

The early age at which the condition emerges means that we must consider not only the importance of correcting the malocclusion, but also evaluate the therapeutic means to be used on such young patients with the aim of restoring masticatory function and balancing growth. Obviously, *the most physiological therapeutic treatment must be sought, one which avoids any traumatic effects*.

Given the complexity of the cranial structure, in the early stages, the side effects are unpredictable and non-preventable; if positional or functional unilateral posterior crossbite is not corrected, owing to its worsening status, the structures will be encouraged by the functional asymmetry into growing asymmetrically and thus, over time, *the condition evolves into a dento-alveolar crossbite*.

4.3.3.2 Dento-alveolar crossbite (Figure 4.11)

In dentoalveolar crossbite, *the position of maximum intercuspation becomes increasingly asymmetric* and the deflected contact from centered position to maximum intercuspation reduces gradually and may be minimal or totally absent: the mandible is definitely off center.

This condition generally affects patients in a later stage of growth, during the period of mixed dentition, as compared with those with functional or positional crossbite. *Dento-alveolar occlusion and tissue support are asymmetric, just like the masticatory function*.

The first period of mixed dentition is very important from a developmental and functional point of view and is characterized by huge changes. The permanent incisors and the first permanent molars erupt in a flat deciduous occlusal plane associated with an immature TMJ. They

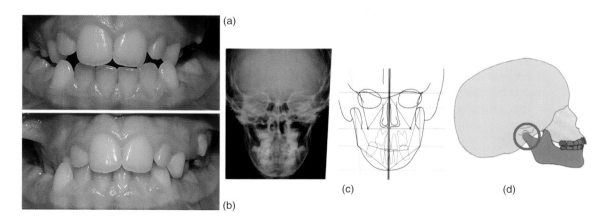

(a)

(c)　　　　　　(d)

(b)

Figure 4.11 Dento-alveolar crossbite: occlusion in maximum intercuspation (b); observe that the centered position is highly unstable (a). Postero-anterior cephalometry (c: frontal plane): both in intercuspation and centered position basal asymmetries are detectable; the dentoalveolar bone is clearly involved. Representation of the mixed dentition stage of development (d: sagittal plane): the TMJ and the mandibular bone are growing; if a posterior crossbite is still present in the mouth of the child, all the basal structures grow in an asymmetric way. This is compensation, not adaptation. See terminology. *Source:* The representation of the mixed dentition stage has been redrawn from Slavicek (2002). Reproduced with permission from R. Slavicek.

are rigid structures and represent interferences in a system free to move. The lingual concavity of the upper new incisors, and not their long axis, represents the anterior limitation of the functional space. The adaptation happens first muscularly and then structurally, resulting in an increased steepness of the articular eminence. The TMJ adapts to different function and occlusion, being characterized by an adaptive type of growth (Thilander *et al.*, 1976; Hinton, 1981).

The first molars are involved in the growth of the posterior regions of the upper maxilla in the three planes of space and in the protrusion of the mandible that stimulates the growth of the mandible. The accurate observation of the molar relationship in this stage of growth is very important for the development of the main function of the stomatognathic system. If the molar relationship is altered, both on the frontal and sagittal planes, functional compensations will occur and asymmetric growth will evolve.

The appropriate orthodontic therapy of dento-alveolar crossbite requires the same features as that for a positional crossbite condition, but the duration of therapy is generally longer because growth and asymmetries are more advanced in comparison with the period of deciduous dentition.

Dento-alveolar crossbite can be seen as a transition phase between the first stages of functional crossbite and the final, irreversible stage. Treatment must be aimed at restoring the correct mandibular position as well as the development of the upper maxilla as soon as possible, and certainly before the pubertal growth spurt.

4.3.3.3 Dento-alveolar–basal crossbite (Figure 4.12)

As time passes, all the structures of the stomatognathic system become asymmetric, involving, in different ways, the posture also. At the end of growth the various districts compensate (adapts in a pathological way see "Terminology") each other and the correction of the unilateral posterior crossbite becomes very difficult or impossible or unsuitable (depending on the individual case), to correct with orthodontic appliances. Of course, it is of utmost importance to always carry out a comprehensive diagnosis complete with precise familial evaluation in order to forecast the potential growth as accurately as possible and identify the most appropriate treatment. From a diagnostic point of view, the photographs of the parents and grandparents are of help in these cases.

However, the dental asymmetry influences the basal asymmetry, via the function, that evolves over time during growth, worsening until adulthood, when it is eventually irreversible and the structures stabilized in asymmetric form.

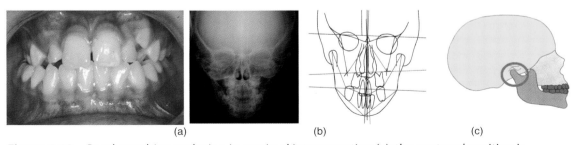

(a)   (b)   (c)

Figure 4.12   Basal crossbite: occlusion in maximal intercuspation (a); the centered position is not detectable. Postero-anterior cephalometry (b: frontal plane): the asymmetries are evident. Representation of the permanent dentition stage of development (c: sagittal plane): at the end of growth the compensatory, basal asymmetries to the posterior crossbite malocclusion are irreversible. *Source:* The representation of the permanent dentition has been redrawn from Slavicek (2002). Reproduced with permission from R. Slavicek.

4.4 Alteration to masticatory function in unilateral posterior crossbite (Figure 4.13)

Following the earlier descriptions of dental and structural characteristics as well as of the development of unilateral posterior crossbite, we will now look at the alterations to masticatory function caused by this type of malocclusion. A number of authors (Lewin, 1985; Ben-Bassat *et al.*, 1993; Throckmorton *et al.*, 2001; Piancino *et al.*, 2006b; Sever *et al.*, 2011) have demonstrated that children with unilateral posterior crossbite display modified chewing patterns on the crossbite side during mastication, characterized by a significant increase in the frequency of reverse-sequence chewing patterns, which refers to movement of the mandible during the closing phase of chewing.

4.4.1 Avoiding biases

Before describing and studying the reverse-sequence chewing cycle, we would like to clarify some biases unfortunately published in the literature.

We have already described how the first instrumental studies of mastication in humans began during the 1960s. One of the most important authors in the field, Ahlgren, traced and recorded mastication using cinematographic methods; by observing the phenomenon carefully he was able to describe seven types of chewing patterns, one of which he defined as a "reverse chewing stroke," where the word *reverse* referred to an exchange of the opening and closing strokes in the frontal plane; that is, when the closing is more lateral than the opening, but the normal direction of closure is maintained. This type of pattern may happen in little children during the earliest growth phases, as Lundeen and Gibbs (1982) described, probably due to the immaturity of the TMJ associated with a flat occlusal plane. Later, Lewin (1985) defined a reverse-sequence chewing cycle as one that is characterized by a reverse closing direction, very different from the exchange of the opening with the closing tracings in the frontal plane.

The use of the word *reverse* with different definitions led to a bias in modern literature, which we would like to resolve before beginning our description of this masticatory condition. Unfortunately, an error of interpretation due to this use of the same term with different meanings resulted in the publication of an article entitled "Is the reverse cycle during chewing abnormal in children with primary dentition?" (Saitoh *et al.*, 2010) in which reference was made to Ahlgren's type 5 cycle (typical of children in the early stages of development). Ahlgren's (1967) use of the term *reverse* relates to the inverted positions of opening and closing strokes; it has no connection whatsoever with the inversion of closing directions, which is instead typical of crossbite as described by Lewin and later confirmed in the literature.

Lewin's definition of a reverse-sequence cycle is that adopted by this current research work and all the international literature (Throckmorton *et al.*, 2001; Piancino *et al.*, 2006b; Sever *et al.*, 2011). It is an important and reliable indicator regarding mastication, both from kinematic and EMG points of view, which has been proven and regularly confirmed. It is our hope that this concept is now clear for reviewers of the scientific journals in the field too.

Before describing the features of reverse-sequence chewing cycles in depth, we would like to underline again that the unilateral posterior crossbite is a malocclusion that may develop in an extremely early phase of development, in deciduous and mixed dentition. The data reported in this chapter arrive from research conducted on individuals in the evolutionary phase, before and after orthognathodontic corrective treatment, in deciduous and mixed dentition. *The role of the teeth is fundamental in masticatory function, whether they be deciduous or permanent. From a functional point of view, a child's deciduous teeth have the same importance as permanent teeth in an adult* – these rigid structures play a determining functional role, and, when dealing with young patients, attention should be paid not only to preventive measures but also to evolutionary control of the condition. We know, in fact, that in some cases permanent teeth may erupt again in crossbite at a later point in time; this has to be considered not a relapse, but the evolution of a complex malocclusion. For this reason, regular monitoring is important, and early corrective measures will prevent the introduction of functional alterations. In other words, we must not reason simply in general terms of teeth but with a functional approach, recognizing that teeth are a means to an end, a way to restore balanced function.

To understand masticatory function from a clinical point of view, it is not enough to know the pattern in absolute terms; we also need to link it between the two sides. For this reason, the section is organized in the following way:

- Section 4.4.2 studies the reverse-sequence chewing pattern and alteration of neuromuscular coordination during chewing on the crossbite side.
- Section 4.4.3 studies the bilateral chewing function (on the crossbite and non-crossbite sides), and the clinical effects of this malocclusion on the function.
- Section 4.4.4 studies the bilateral chewing function before and after orthognathodontic treatment to know the effects of treatment on the function.

4.4.2 The study of masticatory function during chewing on the crossbite side

4.4.2.1 The reverse chewing pattern (Figure 4.14)

The reverse chewing pattern is characterized by the inversion of the closing direction in the last stage of the chewing cycle, which then is defined as a "reverse chewing cycle."

When a unilateral posterior crossbite is present, the number of reverse chewing cycles increases significantly during mastication on the crossbite side in comparison with normal physiological occlusion. Reverse patterns may be present in small numbers also in physiologically conditions, and represent a form of abnormal cycle that may be due (for example) to an attempt to recapture the bolus. Such abnormal cycles cannot be considered part of the regular pattern (i.e., of the patient's motor memory of mastication). When the number of reverse-sequence patterns increases, they become more significant in the patient's mastication, influencing it unequivocally and establishing clinical consequences. Thus, a reverse-sequence chewing cycle is not pathognomonic of crossbite, *but when it emerges often, in significant percentages, then it constitutes an unequivocal clinical indicator of crossbite.*

The closing direction, as described in Chapter 2, is the vector of the closing pattern in the last stage of the chewing cycle. As already stated, the direction of closure in physiological occlusion is linked to the side of mastication (i.e., the bolus side), displaying a clockwise direction when the bolus is between the right-hand hemiarches and an anti-clockwise direction when the bolus is between the left-hand hemiarches. This means that, in cases of right-hand side crossbite, during mastication on the right the chewing cycle displays an anti-clockwise closing direction as opposed to the clockwise direction to be found in physiological conditions. On the contrary, in cases of crossbite on the left-hand side, during mastication on the left the closing direction will be clockwise instead of anti-clockwise.

In healthy conditions of occlusion and mastication, during opening the mandible shifts laterally from the bolus side; then, during closure, it shifts medially via the trans-cuspal and intercuspal stages of mastication opposing the occlusal tooth surfaces. *During a reverse-sequence chewing cycle, the mandible shifts first medially and then laterally, in order to deal with the opposite occluding surfaces of the teeth in crossbite.* The reverse-sequence chewing cycle is set and maintained by the automatisms of the central nervous system's motor control on the basis of peripheral inputs arriving from the periodontal mechanoreceptors (Lund and Kolta, 2006; Morquette et al., 2012).

The reverse closing direction is not an isolated sign, but it is an indicator of *altered pattern* and is linked with other irregularities:

1. morphological changes;
2. changes to the pattern position in space.

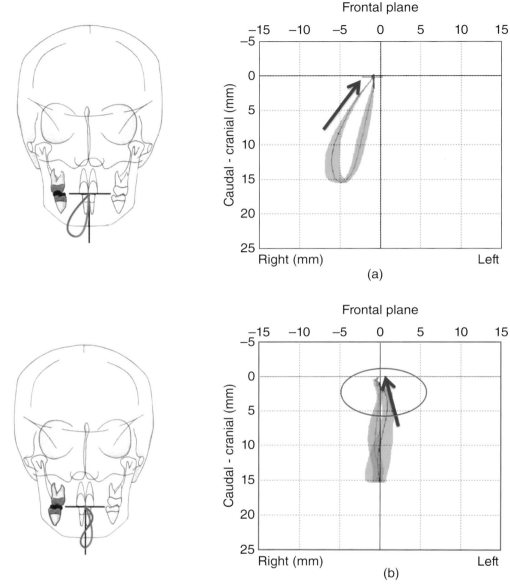

Figure 4.13 Physiological (a) versus reverse (b) chewing pattern during chewing on the right side.

1. The alterations that occur when closing direction is reversed are of a morphological and positional nature. The morphology of a reverse-sequence chewing pattern differs in that it may feature *crossovers between the opening and closing tracks* – this may occur once or more during the same cycle or the tracks may never cross over, as the cycle is totally reversed. In this case, to an untrained eye, the pattern may appear normal, but in reality, due to the reverse closing direction, the chewing cycle dynamic is entirely altered (Figure 4.14c). What

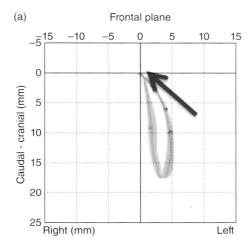

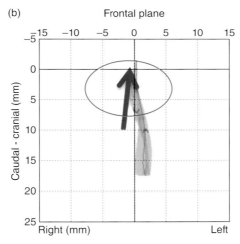

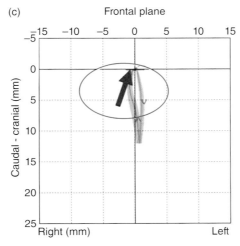

Figure 4.14 Physiological (a) pattern versus different type of reverse chewing cycles, with (b) and without (c) crossover of the tracings, during chewing on the left side.

distinguishes a reverse chewing cycle (with or without crossovers) from a normal physio-logical cycle *is the reduced distance between the opening and closing tracks*, which makes the chewing cycle *"tight" and repetitive* (Piancino *et al.*, 2009). Some authors have also proven a *reduced maximum opening track during reverse-sequence chewing cycles* (Throckmorton *et al.*, 2001).

2. In addition to the morphological alterations, when the closing direction is reversed, there is an abnormal position of the cycle in space, which develops very near to the vertical axis or the opposite side to the bolus. Thus, the area between the opening and closing tracks of reverse-sequence chewing cycles is slighter than normal and develops along the vertical axis, or on the contralateral side, instead of on the bolus side as generally occurs in healthy occlusion.

Consequently, the closing angle indicates that the final stage of the closing track is very close to the vertical axis (i.e. the closing direction is reverse). *The verticality of the closing angle, the reduced distance between the opening and closing tracks, and the evolution of the pattern on the contralateral as opposed to the bolus side* are typical features of reverse-sequence chewing cycles and are all *indicators of reduced masticatory efficiency* (Wilding and Lewin, 1994). The efficiency of the chewing cycles during the developmental age is important for the correlated vectorial forces that represent the functional matrix and the stimulus to the bone growth. Masticatory function is very important for the maxillary growth (see Chapter 3, Section 3.9 and Figure 3.20). The change of vectors and reduction of forces during development will have an impact on the growing structure (Thilander *et al.*, 1976; Kiliaridis *et al.*, 1999; Thilander, 1995). The alterations to the pattern described here are clear, easy to recognize and diagnose, and constitute clinical importance that we will hereafter explain. Thus, we will tackle "masticatory function" and not merely individual cycles, in order to understand the clinical implications.

The number of reverse-sequence chewing cycles during mastication on the crossbite side is extremely high, cited in the literature as being between 40 and 70% on average (depending on the severity of the malocclusion and on bolus type). In fact, *the percentage of reverse-sequence cycles is significantly higher during mastication of hard boluses as opposed to soft ones* (Piancino *et al.*, 2006bb) and *this increases according to the number of teeth involved in the crossbite condition in the posterior regions* (Lewin, 1985). In any case, the number of reverse-sequence cycles in cases of unilateral posterior crossbite where the first molar only is involved is still significantly higher than in patients without a crossbite condition. *Careful attention must always be paid to those cases of patients with one (molar) or multiple teeth involved in crossbite, both during treatment and during the follow-up period*, as motor memory requires time to change in a stable way and the risk of a return to the malocclusion state is real.

However, unilateral posterior crossbite of one tooth generally involves the first permanent molar, which emerges at around 6 years of age. The first permanent molar is the tooth that is most concerned with mastication and early treatment of this molar is very important for establishing a balance function. Furthermore, at around 6 years of age, children are in a transitional period, midway between deciduous and permanent dentition. This is a period of huge change in occlusion and structural and neuromuscular elements, meaning that the restoration of healthy function is essential for the future efficiency of the stomatognathic system. The early correction of unilateral posterior crossbite involves the entire masticatory function and is of huge importance for the health and balanced growth of the stomatognathic system even when just the first permanent molar is involved.

4.4.2.2 *Alteration of neuromuscular coordination between sides during reverse-sequence chewing pattern* (Figures 4.15, 4.16, and 4.17)

Following the same reasoning as before, and in light of the fact that mastication is a rhythmic movement controlled and maintained by the automatisms of the central nervous system for the coordination of masticatory muscles, we would expect a reverse-sequence chewing cycle to be

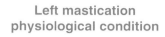

**Left mastication
physiological condition**

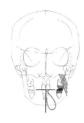

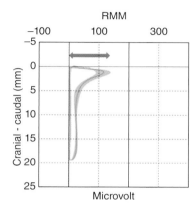

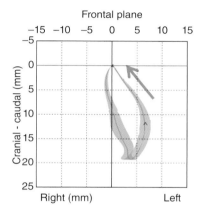

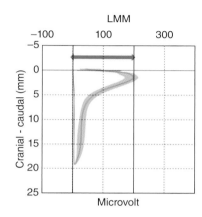

**Left mastication
crossbite condition**

**Altered muscular
coordination**

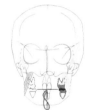

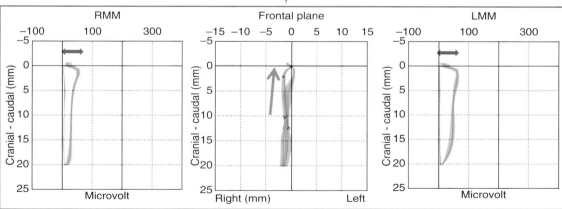

Figure 4.15 Comparison between physiological (*top*) activation of masseters during chewing on the left side and altered coordination during reverse chewing cycles on the left crossbite side (*bottom*).

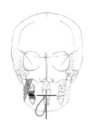

Right mastication physiological condition

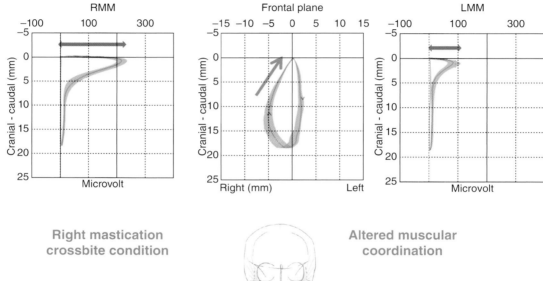

Right mastication crossbite condition

Altered muscular coordination

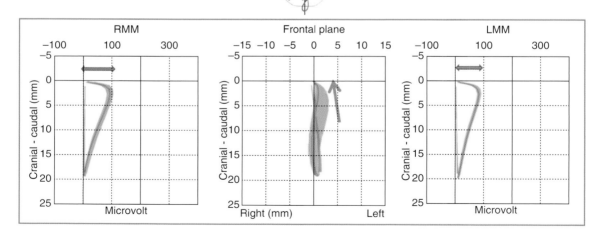

Figure 4.16 Comparison between physiological (*top*) activation of masseters during chewing on the right side and altered coordination during reverse chewing cycles on the right crossbite side (*bottom*). Green tracings: opening; red tracings: closing.

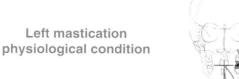

Left mastication
physiological condition

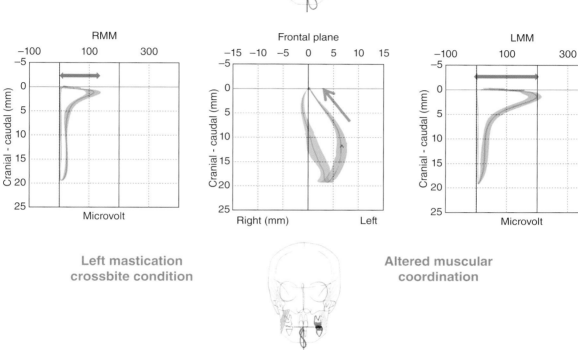

Left mastication
crossbite condition

Altered muscular
coordination

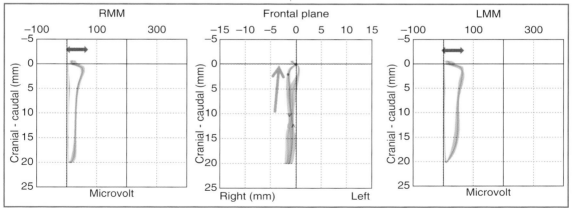

Figure 4.17 Comparison between physiological (*top*) activation of masseters during chewing on the left side and altered coordination during reverse chewing cycles on the left crossbite side (*bottom*).

flanked by neuromuscular activity that is different to that of normal physiological conditions (Katoh *et al.*, 1982; Lund *et al.*, 1999; Yoshino *et al.*, 1999; Ishii *et al.*, 2002; Johnsen and Trulsson, 2003). Let us remember that, in normal healthy occlusion, the masseter on the bolus side displays an EMG almost twice as wide as that of the contralateral masseter. *As mastication is a rhythmic and alternate movement, this coordination between the two masseters is important in maintaining its equilibrium and for harmonious growth of the stomatognathic system.* In cases of crossbite, it has been shown that a *reverse-sequence chewing cycle* that develops during mastication on the crossbite side *displays a much smaller EMG amplitude of the masseter on the crossbite side as opposed to physiological occlusion and to that on the contralateral side.* Furthermore, the latter displays a width in accordance with the increase in compensation. In other words, the masseter of the crossbite side is always hypoactive in comparison with the masseter on the healthy side. It is clear that there is an *alteration of normal masseter activation between the bolus side and the contralateral side during mastication on the crossbite side* (Piancino *et al.*, 2009).

As far as temporal indicators are concerned, it has been shown that there is a reduction in the time spent on functional maximum intercuspation between one cycle and another during mastication on the crossbite side as opposed to the healthy side (Piancino *et al.*, 2009; Sever *et al.*, 2011) and a reduction in the average occlusal pause phase of all mastication; that is, the time between the end of one chewing cycle and the beginning of the opening phase of the next cycle. For these reasons, the reverse-sequence chewing cycle may be termed as a "dis-kinetic" type, in the sense that it loses its normal kinetic features and neuromuscular coordination, with alterations to its EMG amplitude and activated/silent times between one cycle and another. These features are in agreement with the parameters of reduced masticatory efficiency of the reverse chewing patterns

4.4.3 The study of mastication during chewing on the crossbite and non-crossbite side; effects of asymmetry of the malocclusion on function

4.4.3.1 Bilateral chewing patterns in unilateral posterior crossbite malocclusion

As described in Chapter 2, one of the key points of mastication in patients with physiological occlusion is the production of specular and symmetrical chewing patterns. We know that patients with unilateral posterior crossbite display irregular chewing cycles and altered muscular activation when chewing on the affected side, with a much higher percentage of reverse-sequence cycles and the loss of neuromuscular coordination, as described earlier. *However, to understand well the clinical consequences of the crossbite condition, we must look at "masticatory function" and not just at single cycles.* Thus, the question is: What happens to the chewing pattern during mastication on the healthy side?

We know that when chewing takes place on the crossbite side the number of reverse-sequence chewing cycles significantly increases, but what happens to the chewing cycle on the healthy side? The literature (Throckmorton *et al.*, 2001; Piancino *et al.*, 2006b; Sever *et al.*, 2011) states that the chewing pattern during mastication on the healthy side maintains the same characteristics as physiological mastication; in other words, not only is the closing direction normal (clockwise during mastication on the right, anti-clockwise during mastication on the left), but the pattern morphology in terms of closure angle, height, width, and spatial position also displays no significant differences from that of mastication in a patient with physiological occlusion (Figures 4.18 and 4.19).

The reverse-sequence chewing cycle, then, occurs only on the crossbite side, whilst *the chewing cycle displays the normal physiological closing direction on the healthy side.* This fact is extremely important from a clinical point of view as it is the reason why unilateral posterior crossbite is characterized not only by dental asymmetry but also, and above all, by *functional asymmetry.*

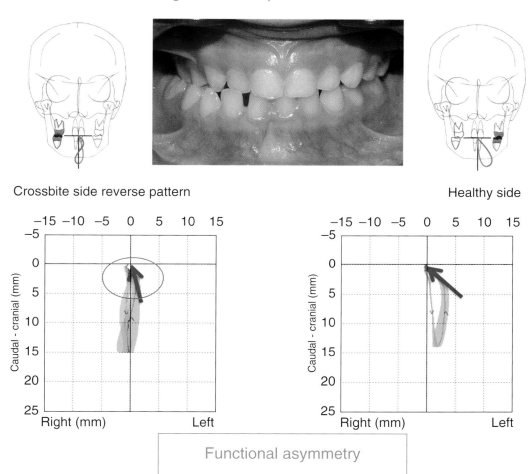

Figure 4.18 Chewing patterns during chewing on the right crossbite side and on the left non-crossbite side. Observe the functional asymmetry of the chewing pattern and the reverse anomalous pattern on the crossbite side. Green tracings: opening; red tracings: closing.

We published an article on this very subject, in collaboration with A. Lewin, proving what he himself clearly explained about reverse-sequence chewing cycles in conditions of unilateral posterior crossbite (Lewin, 1985; Piancino et al., 2006b). The results of this study showed that the percentage of reverse-sequence chewing cycles during mastication on the crossbite side in children aged between 7 and 11 years old is significantly higher than the number of reverse cycles on the healthy side, both with a soft bolus ($P = 0.0003$) and with a hard bolus ($P = 0.0003$). The percentage of reverse-sequencing chewing cycles was 41% (0–96%) for a soft bolus and 66% (0–98%) for a hard bolus when chewing on the crossbite side and 5% (0–31%) for both a soft and a hard bolus when chewing on the non-crossbite side. This high statistical frequency shows that we have identified a functional phenomenon, which may be viewed as a highly reliable valid indicator for the monitoring of masticatory function. However, the *muscular activity is the element that can most serve to explain the consequences for skeletal*

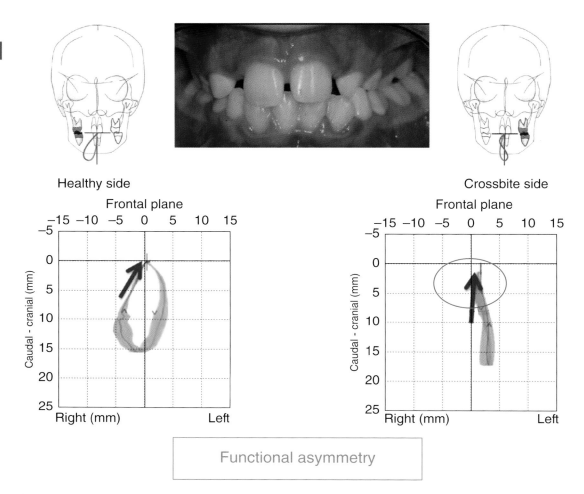

Figure 4.19 Chewing patterns during chewing on the right non-crossbite side and on the left crossbite side. Observe the functional asymmetry of the chewing pattern and the reverse anomalous pattern on the crossbite side. Green tracings: opening; red tracings: closing.

growth and the collateral effects of the malocclusion on the entire stomatognathic system. So, let us analyze the bilateral muscular activation to understand the clinical consequences of this malocclusion on growth and balance.

4.4.3.2 Bilateral neuromuscular coordination in unilateral posterior crossbite malocclusion (Figure 4.20)

The modification of reverse-sequence chewing cycles, which we described earlier in terms of morphological pattern, distribution of the cycles in space, and so on, is accompanied by an alteration in neuromuscular coordination that leads to an imbalance of the masseter muscles during mastication on the crossbite side, as described in Section 4.4.2. We already know that the chewing pattern shows normal characteristics on the healthy side.

4.4.3.2.1 What happens to the muscular coordination during chewing on the normal side?

The physiological pattern on the healthy side is assisted by normal healthy activation and coordination of the masseter muscles.

We performed a kinematic and EMG study of this question, regarding both reverse- and non-reverse-sequence chewing cycles in patients with unilateral posterior crossbite (Piancino *et al.*, 2009). The results showed that the percentage difference in masseter amplitude on the two sides is significantly different during chewing on the crossbite side compared with chewing on the healthy side. The masseter on the crossbite side was hypoactive in comparison with the healthy side, whilst the masseter of the healthy side displayed hyperactive characteristics in relative compensation. In agreement with these results, the literature reveals, from an anatomical point of view, *a significant difference in volume* between the masseter on the crossbite side and that on the healthy side in a group of children aged between 7 and 11 years old with unilateral posterior crossbite (Kiliaridis *et al.*, 2007). The reduced volume of the masseter on the crossbite side is an anatomic consequence of the masticatory functional imbalance, characterized not only by a decrease in EMG amplitude of the muscle on the crossbite side but also by a relative increase in EMG activity in the muscle on the healthy side. We must add, to clarify the features of neuromuscular control, that the dominance of the masseter on the bolus side (whether this be the crossbite or healthy side) is maintained throughout. Thus, in the event of severe discoordination between one side and the other, which may lead to muscle hypotrophy on the crossbite side and compensatory muscle hypertrophy on the healthy side, the underlying bilateral neuromuscular control is still maintained. However, the variation in muscular activation between one side and the other is the basis of that functional asymmetry which is typical of unilateral posterior crossbite. *The altered muscular activation corresponds to the altered kinematics of the reverse chewing cycles that can be considered an indicator of the functional asymmetry.*

Remembering that this malocclusion occurs at a very early stage in development, during primary dentition, and can involve permanent dentition at a later stage, it is clear that the functional asymmetry described will have a biological impact on the growing structures, leading to asymmetric anatomical structures (bones, TMJ, muscles, and teeth) on completion of growth. Such asymmetries may be prevented by non-traumatic orthodontic therapy even at a very early stage in development aimed to restore the balance of neuromuscular activation during masticatory function.

4.4.3.2.2 The question of the preferential side of mastication

At this point we would like to tackle the question of the preferential side of mastication, an issue that has often been discussed on an international level. Muscular asymmetry that develops at an *early age* in patients with unilateral posterior crossbite is caused by *alterations to the neuromuscular coordination resulting from the malocclusion*, and, usually, not by any presumed preferential side of mastication. As proven by different authors, there is not a preferential side of mastication in children with crossbite conditions (Egermark-Eriksson *et al.*, 1990; Martín *et al.*, 2000; Andrade *et al.*, 2010). A preferential side of mastication may appear in later stages of development and it may not hold a direct link with occlusal contact areas (Wilding and Lewin, 1994). Articular asymmetry which arises during development as a result of the malocclusion (Pirttiniemi *et al.*, 1990, 1991) may lead to a preferential side of mastication in adulthood (Santana-Mora *et al.*, 2013) and cause further deterioration to the asymmetry at that time (Thilander and Bjerklin, 2012).

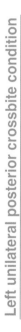

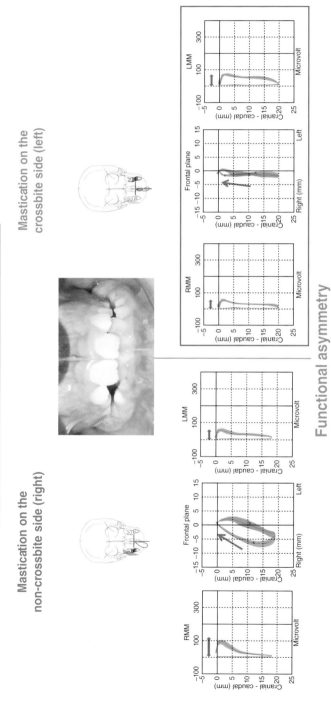

Figure 4.20 Bilateral chewing patterns and EMG activation of the masseters during chewing on the right non-crossbite side and on the left crossbite side. Observe the functional asymmetry of the chewing pattern and the EMG asymmetrical activation between sides. Green tracings: opening; red tracings: closing.

4.4.3.3 Molecular aspects and magnetic resonance imaging of the masseter related to the asymmetry of the muscular activation

Knowing the special characteristics of the masseter muscle previously described in Chapter 3, the functional asymmetry shown by the EMG recordings during chewing in unilateral posterior crossbite conditions has raised the question of whether the composition of the integrin and sarcoglycan network of the masseter could be related to the functional aspects (Cutroneo *et al.*, 2012).

Integrins are a family of heterodimeric cell surface membrane proteins that mediate the interaction of cells with extracellular matrix proteins and with additional molecules during their environment. These proteins also provide a bi-directional signaling between the extracellular matrix and the cytoplasm and in the signaling with the cell matrix. Integrins also play a key role in cell adhesion, including intercellular interactions, and, therefore, they are involved in various biological phenomena, such as cell migration, differentiation, tissues repair, and programmed cell death. Thus, it is known that integrins are receptors of the cellular surface composed of two associated subunits α and β and that more than 20 different integrin transmembrane receptors have been described up to the present; α_7B and β_1D are the predominant integrins in adult skeletal muscle.

Each integrin is composed of a noncovalent linking between α and β subunits. In particular, the $\alpha_7\beta_1$-integrin is concentrated at neuromuscular and myotendinous junctions, and it is located along the sarcolemma at costameres with an important role in the functions of the skeletal muscle. It was demonstrated that congenital myopathies are caused by mutations in the human integrin α_7 gene (*ITGA7*), confirming the importance of the $\alpha_7\beta_1$-integrin in maintaining normal skeletal muscle physiology.

The β_1A isoform is abundantly expressed in proliferating myogenic precursor cells, but during myodifferentiation it is replaced by the β_1D isoform. In mature skeletal muscle, β_1A is expressed only at a low level, if at all, whereas the predominant β_1D becomes concentrated in the sarcolemma of myotendinous junctions, neuromuscular junctions, and costameres. It was demonstrated that a bi-directional signaling between integrins and sarcoglycans exists in order to regulate the biological function of the muscle fibers.

Regarding this, it is important to comprehend that the sarcoglycan subcomplex (SGC) is a well-known system of interaction between extracellular matrix and sarcolemma-associated cytoskeleton in skeletal and cardiac muscle. Sarcoglycans play a key role in the pathogenesis of many muscular dystrophies, such as Duchenne and Becker muscular dystrophies and sarcoglycanopathies. In fact, recent developments in molecular genetics have demonstrated that mutation in each of the single sarcoglycan genes 17q, 4q, 13q, and 5q causes a series of recessive autosomal dystrophin-positive muscular dystrophies, not accompanied by a lack of dystrophin, called sarcoglycanopathies or limb girdle muscular dystrophies (LGMD types 2D, 2E, 2C, and 2F respectively).

The SGC consists of four transmembrane proteins: α-SG, specifically expressed in skeletal and cardiac muscle; β-SG, most abundant in cardiac and skeletal muscle, but also expressed in placenta, kidney, liver, and lung; and γ- and δ-SG, which are highly similar among themselves and similar to β-SG.

Whereas δ-SG is detected in all types of muscle, γ-SG is expressed exclusively in striated muscle. Attempts to immunolocalize γ-SG in smooth muscle have failed, and the question of whether γ-SG or a smooth muscle isoform exists is unanswered, although previous reports anticipated the presence of γ-SG in smooth muscle. A fifth sarcoglycan subunit, ε-SG, is more broadly expressed, showing a wider tissue distribution. Despite its homology to α-SG and its presence in skeletal muscle, endogenous ε-SG is unable to rescue phenotypes associated with α-SG loss.

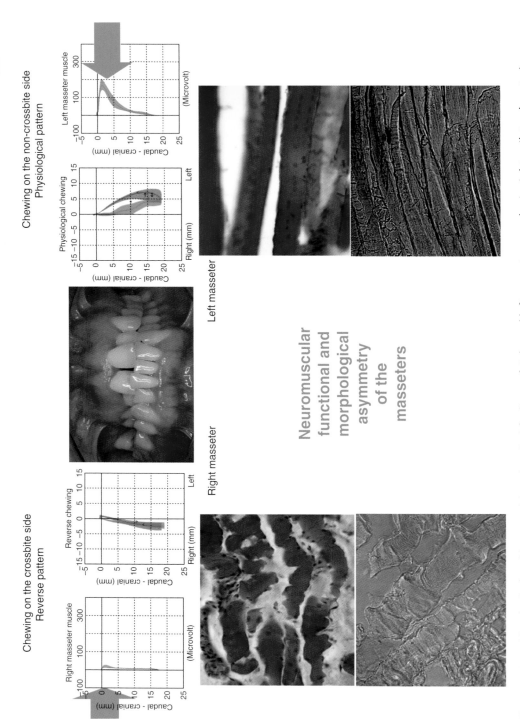

Figure 4.21 Histological and immunohistochemical findings of right and left masseter muscles in right unilateral posterior crossbite. The muscular alterations on the crossbite side (right side) are evident. Green tracings: opening; red tracings: closing. *Source*: G. Cutroneo, University of Messina, Messina, Italy. Reproduced with permission from G. Cutroneo.

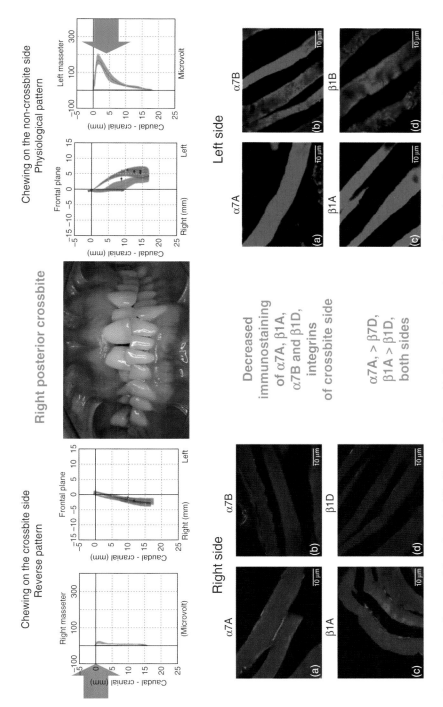

Figure 4.22 Immunohistochemical findings of right and left masseter muscles in right unilateral posterior crossbite using antibodies against sarcoglycans. The increased staining patterns of sarcoglycans on the crossbite side (right side) are evident. Green tracings: opening; red tracings: closing. *Source:* G. Cutroneo, University of Messina, Messina, Italy. Reproduced with permission from G. Cutroneo.

Interestingly, previous studies on chimpanzee have demonstrated that in the masseter of alpha males the α_7A and β_1A integrins were clearly increased compared with α_7B and β_1D, which are usually more expressed in other striated muscles (Favaloro *et al.*, 2009).

Thus, considering the important function of the masseter muscle, its particular role in chewing cycles, and its serious EMG alterations in unilateral posterior crossbite malocclusions, we studied this muscle in order to verify its composition in the integrin network. Using immunohistochemical and molecular techniques, we analyzed human masseter muscles of surgical patients affected by severe class III malocclusion, associated with right unilateral posterior crossbite, to comprehend the role of integrins in these masticatory muscles. The study was conducted, on the basis of the EMG results, in collaboration with the maxillofacial surgery division of the University of Turin (Professor G. Ramieri) and with the University of Messina (Professor G. Anastasi and Professorr G. Cutroneo) for the morphological and molecular analysis.

The results showed that the amount of integrins appeared to be significantly lower on the crossbite side than that detected on the non-crossbite side. But the most important finding is that β_1A appeared clearly present in adult masseter muscle and that α_7A and β_1A isoforms (the isoforms usually present during development, but not in the adult striated muscle) were predominant in both masseters in comparison with the α_7B and β_1D isoforms (typical of adult striated muscle) respectively (Figures 4.21 and 4.22).

All integrins decreased in the crossbite side in comparison with the non-crossbite side. Also, in the side not affected by crossbite, integrins were significantly increased.

Our present findings analyzing the pattern of the integrins in masseter muscle showed that the integrins play a key role not only in the muscular activity but also in the optimization of contractile forces of this muscle.

Within the same research, histological and immunohistochemical findings of the masseters showed disrupted fibers and significant low nuclei concentration on the crossbite compared to the non-crossbite side (Figure 4.21).

Finally, in agreement with these results, thanks to the collaborative partnership between Prof. P. Bramanti IRCCS Centro Neurolesi "Bonino Pulejo" Messina–Italy, recent studies on patients with unilateral posterior crossbite diseases, conducted by tractography obtained by a modern imaging technique – the diffusion tense magnetic resonance scan – not only confirmed the lower volume of the masseter on the crossbite side, but have revealed an irregular remodeling of the same muscle (Figure 4.23).

This result could be due to the particular composition of masseter, since it contains hybrid fibers showing the capacity to modify the contractile properties to optimize the energy efficiency or the action of the muscle during contraction. Moreover, masseter is characterized by a high turnover of muscle fibers producing a regeneration process. This may indicate a longer time to heal, justifying the loss of β_1D and the consequential increase of β_1A. Thus, our data provide the first suggestion that integrins in masseter muscle play a key role regulating the functional activity of muscle and allowing the optimization of contractile forces. This result could be considered the molecular aspect of the functional and neuromuscular control in unilateral posterior crossbites.

4.4.3.4 *Clinical aspects of the asymmetry of the muscular activation*

Such an asymmetric masticatory function, established in the early stages of development, has an undeniable biological impact on the developing structures, as has been repeatedly underlined in the literature (Pirttiniemi *et al.*, 1990; Poikela *et al.*, 1997; Pinto *et al.*, 2001; Sonnesen *et al.*, 2001; Thilander and Bjerklin, 2012), and results at the end of growth in asymmetric anatomical structures (bones, TMJ, muscles, and teeth) that can no longer be corrected by orthognathodontic intervention. This irreversibility is due to the asymmetric development of complex skeletal

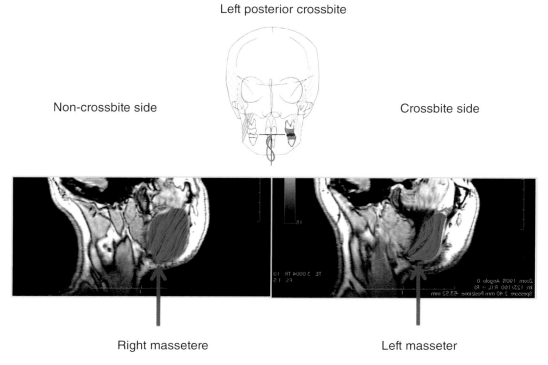

Left posterior crossbite

Non-crossbite side

Crossbite side

Right massetere

Left masseter

Figure 4.23   Tractography of the left and right masseter muscles obtained by diffusion tensor resonance magnetic imaging (DTRMI) scan in a patient with left posterior crossbite malocclusion. Observe the increased volume of the contralateral muscle (right masseter) compared with the crossbite side (left masseter). *Source:* G. Anastasi University of Messina, Messina, Italy. Reproduced with permission of G. Anastasi.

and joint structures that have lower adjustment capacity at the end of the growth development. In addition, the motor memory has adapted to peripheral inputs during this period and has become extremely resistant to change (Throckmorton *et al.*, 2001). In clinical practice, we know that the prosthetic correction of posterior crossbites may result in a functional disturbance that is often unbearable for the patient, lasting until the dental prosthesis breaks.

It is important to understand the neuromuscular asymmetry of the masticatory function of unilateral posterior crossbite in order to understand the origin of the clinical effects of malocclusion and the need for early treatment (Thilander *et al.*, 1984; Pirttiniemi *et al.*, 1990, 1991; Thilander and Lennartsson, 2002). In fact, mastication is a movement that is repeated many times during the course of the day, every day, and in normal healthy conditions it stimulates the growth of the stomatognathic system structures, especially facial sutures, in a harmonious and symmetric manner. The role of masticatory force is important in structural development, as shown in experiments regarding the different developmental process of the median palatine suture and condyle according to bolus types (Engström *et al.*, 1986; Kiliaridis *et al.*, 1999). We have already described the different morphology and vectors of the patterns of a soft bolus as compared with a hard bolus, the latter being characterized by higher width and height, a wider angle of closure, greater lateral shift, and higher EMG amplitude. On the basis of the fact that forces and vectors represent the functional matrix, which is the stimulus to the bone growth, there is evidence in literature of the influence of the type of bolus on growth. Some studies showed that laboratory animals fed with soft-consistency food developed a much more calcified and much less active palatine suture, as well as a less developed condyle, both in length and width, than animals fed with normal-consistency food (see Chapter 5).

Furthermore, as Slavicek (2002) states, masticatory force is transmitted to the skeletal structures of the splanchnocranium via the dental roots, particularly of the upper first molar. All these data confirm the functional matrix theory of Moss and Enlow, which clearly defines the functional neuromuscular activity role in the structural development of humans (Enlow, 1986). The consequence of unilateral posterior crossbite is a structural asymmetry of the cranial bones that we can clearly detect on the palatal vault of patients with this malocclusion. The hemi-palate on the crossbite side is narrower and less developed than that on the contralateral normal side. It is still not easy to detect the asymmetries of the other cranial bones, but we hope that 3D imaging will evolve in order to improve our knowledge in this field (Frongia *et al.*, 2013). From this, it is also clear that we must instead *evolve entirely in terms of diagnosis, reasoning, mentality, and "orthognathodontic" treatment*, all based on the study and monitoring of the function. Teeth are an important factor but cannot be the only therapeutic focus, as the true objective is functional rebalancing of the stomatognathic system (essential for the future life quality of young patients, but also for adults whose compensation capacities are more limited).

Not all dental malocclusions cause such a severe imbalance of neuromuscular activity. In the case of unilateral posterior crossbite, the involvement of masticatory function is due to the influence of the teeth responsible for bolus grinding in the frontal plane (i.e., molars and premolars). The system compensates (adapts in a pathological way see "Terminology") for dental asymmetry by establishing neuromuscular asymmetry, thus exposing patients with this type of malocclusion to a higher risk (in adulthood) of painful chronic disorders of the cranio-facial region, as recently revised studies have shown (Thilander and Bjerklin, 2012). It is not necessary to wait for complex (almost impossible) longitudinal studies of a human's intrinsic variability or variability over time in order to prove that the stomatognathic system in patients with unilateral posterior crossbite is more at risk of compensatory effects and symptomatic pathologies than patients with symmetric and physiological occlusion. The results described regarding kinematic, muscular, histological, and fMRI diffusion tensor imaging are all in agreement between each other, showing the same results from different points of view (Brin *et al.*, 1996; Onozuka *et al.*, 2002; Piancino *et al.*, 2006b; Piancino *et al.*, 2009; Andrade *et al.*, 2010). When the system becomes decompensated, the removal of etiopathogenetic causes is no longer possible; the etiopathogenesis of the pain, at an advanced stage of imbalance has multiple origins, the appropriate therapy is multidisciplinary, and almost never entirely successful. The only way to halt the inexorable increase of chronic algic pathologies in the facial region of crossbite patients is to prevent them by correcting this malocclusion in the early stages of development with non-traumatic treatment in full respect of physiological conditions and tissue biology in order to reach the healthy functioning of the stomatognathic system.

4.4.4 The study of masticatory function before and after orthognathodontic treatment; effects of therapy on function

4.4.4.1 *Reverse and non-reverse chewing pattern before/after therapy* (Figures 4.24 and 4.25)

After identifying the functional characteristics of crossbite, the research moved on to study the effects on the function after therapy with the function generating bite (FGB) appliance (Bracco and Solinas, 1979). We know that the aim of early therapy is to improve function and growth and that it is of clinical relevance, for successful orthodontic therapy, to consider not only the repositioning of teeth within the dental arches but also the effects of therapy on function.

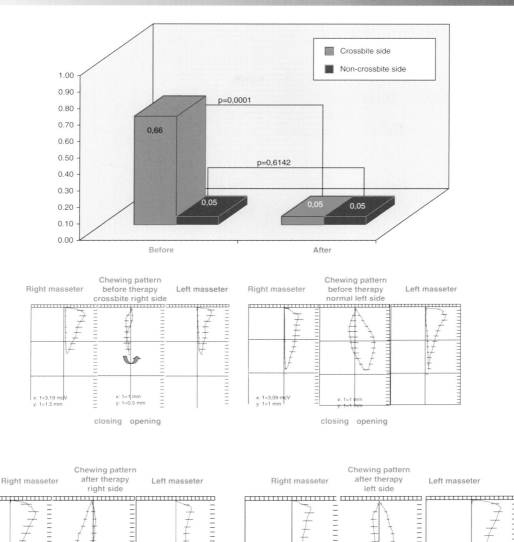

Figure 4.24 *Top:* comparison of percentage of reverse chewing cycles during chewing on the crossbite side and on the healthy side, before and after therapy. *Center:* chewing pattern and EMG activity of a patient with right unilateral posterior crossbite before correction; *bottom:* after correction. Green tracings: opening; red tracings: closing. *Source:* Piancino *et al.* (2006). Reproduced with permission from Oxford University Press.

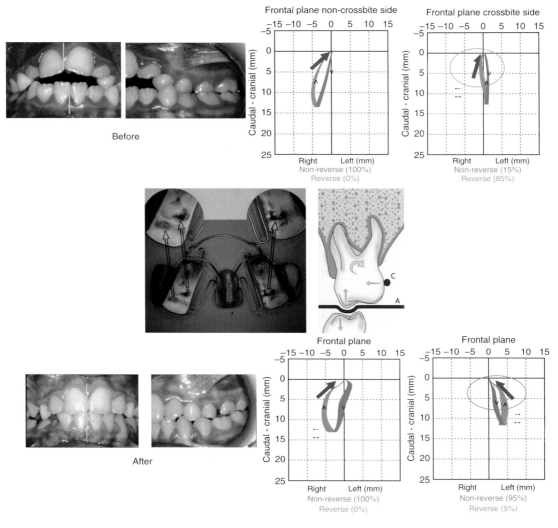

Figure 4.25 Comparison of chewing pattern in left posterior crossbite before and after therapy with function generating bite appliance. Green tracings: opening; red tracings: closing.

As already reported, the prevalence of reverse-sequence chewing cycles before treatment of unilateral posterior crossbite (Piancino *et al.*, 2006b) showed a *significant difference between the percentages of reverse-sequencing chewing patterns on the crossbite and non-crossbite sides*.

After therapy, a statistically significant difference was also found when comparing the percentage of reverse-sequencing chewing patterns before and after therapy on the crossbite side. Before therapy, the percentage of reverse-sequencing chewing cycles was 41% (0–96%) when chewing a soft bolus and 66% (0–98%) when chewing a hard bolus. After therapy, it was 7% (0–59%; $P < 0.001$) and 5% (0–3%; $P < 0.001$) respectively.

No statistically significant difference was observed when the percentages of reverse-sequencing chewing cycles were compared before and after therapy during chewing on the non-crossbite side.

Moreover, what is very important is that any significant difference was observed between sides after therapy, meaning that the functional asymmetry had been restored. The functional appliance successfully achieved the aim of the early therapy to reposition teeth within the dental arches and to improve the balance of the masticatory function.

The restoration of closing direction is the first important change in the chewing cycle achieved with functional therapy. But, as well as monitoring the correction of reverse-sequence chewing cycles, the restoration of muscular activation is very important from a clinical point of view (Piancino *et al.*, 2009, 2015b).

4.4.4.2 The bilateral muscular coordination between sides before and after therapy

The correction of reverse chewing patterns is an important sign because it indicates that the masticatory function is restoring the symmetry of the movement. The kinematics of the mandible could be considered an index of the muscular coordination that is the final aim of our therapy.

In our study we characterized the kinematics and masseter muscle activation in unilateral posterior crossbite. It was concluded that, when chewing on the crossbite side, the masseter activity is reduced on the mastication side (crossbite) and is unaltered (non-reverse cycles) or increased (reverse) on the contralateral side (Piancino *et al.*, 2009). This means that the amount of overload of the nonaffected side depends on the percentage of reverse cycles.

The altered muscular activation corresponds to the altered kinematics of the reverse chewing cycles that can be considered an indicator of the functional asymmetry. The reduction in the percentage of reverse cycles is important for decreasing the altered muscular activity. The lowering of reverse chewing cycles reduces the muscular overload of the non-affected side. A functional correction of the chewing cycles is the real aim of the early orthodontic therapy.

In a recent study, the activation and coordination of the masseter muscles of children with unilateral posterior crossbite were evaluated during chewing of either soft or hard boluses, on both the affected and nonaffected sides, before and after functional therapy with the function generating bite (FGB) appliance. After the intervention, a significant reduction in reverse chewing cycles was observed when chewing on the previous crossbite side ($P < 0.001$) and the angle of closure was no longer different between sides for either bolus type ($P < 0.001$). Furthermore, the percentage difference in masseter muscle activity between sides was similar for the patients after therapy to that of control subjects, thus indicating that the intervention had induced a symmetrization and a favorable change in the neuromuscular control of chewing. This was observed for both bolus types. The normalization of muscle activity between sides after the intervention corresponds to the symmetry observed for the kinematic data post treatment. In particular, the reduction of the percentage of reverse chewing cycles is an important sign of the restoration of the coordination of bilateral masseter muscle activity (Figures 4.24 and 4.26).

These findings indicate that the functional intervention induced a favorable change in the neural control of chewing. From a clinical point of view this is an important result because it demonstrates that the repositioning of teeth within the dental arches obtained with the FGB appliance was matched with recovery of the altered muscular activation between sides, during masticatory function.

To understand these significant results (both in terms of pattern and neuromuscular activity), it is important to explain the type of orthognathodontic appliance used. The appliance used was a functionalizing device, individually manufactured and made of acrylic resin and resilient stainless steel, with posterior metallic bite planes preventing the teeth from

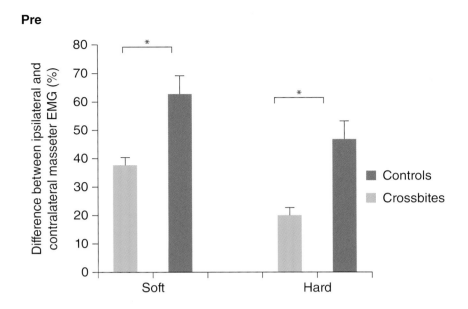

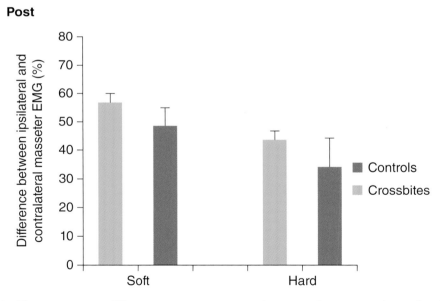

Figure 4.26 The percentage difference in masseter muscle activity between sides in the children with unilateral posterior crossbite (*top*) when chewing on the crossbite side was significantly (*) lower (yellow) compared with the difference observed for the control group (blue), and corresponded to the altered kinematics of the reverse chewing cycles. After therapy (*bottom*) it was similar for patients and controls.

making intercuspal contact. At the end of treatment, the buccal cusps of the upper teeth (which were previously in a crossbite condition) overlapped the lower teeth, thus providing the appropriate physiological stimuli from peripheral receptors and proprioreceptors. The appliance (its components, actions, and effects) will be explained in depth in Chapter 5. At this point we will simply underline that a non-traumatic therapy was carried out, character-ized by the spontaneous repositioning of the mandible in space and controlled dental con-tacts during all stages of the orthodontic movement, with self-regulated, intermittent forces, not imposed and not continuous, in full respect of normal physiological and biological con-ditions of the system.

Some authors have evaluated the alterations of chewing cycles after dental correction of a unilateral posterior crossbite (Ben-Bassat *et al.*, 1993) with fixed appliances, but they did not show any significant change in the masticatory function (Ben-Bassat *et al.*, 1993; Brin *et al.*, 1996; Throckmorton *et al.*, 2001). Throckmorton et al. (2001) evaluated masticatory cycles in children treated with rapid palatal expansion but did not find a reduction in the reverse-sequencing chewing pattern. They speculated that the reverse sequencing persists after dental correction of a unilateral posterior crossbite because this malocclusion develops dur-ing eruption of the primary dentition and has an influence on the developing central pattern generator, establishing the reverse-sequencing type of chewing pattern that is, then, resist-ant to change. Recently, a number of articles have been published evaluating the maximal clenching and/or border movements in unilateral posterior crossbite patients before and before/after correction (Martín *et al.*, 2012) As explained in Chapter 2, masticatory function is not comparable with border movements or maximal clenching, which require different considerations.

As previously explained, because this malocclusion occurs at an early stage in development, it has a significant influence on the developing motor control of mastication in the central nervous system (Throckmorton *et al.*, 2001). Asymmetric masticatory function during growth has a biological impact duing growing and leads to irreversible asymmetric anatomical struc-tures (bones, TMJ, muscles, and teeth) on completion of growth (Enlow, 1986; Pirttiniemi *et al.* 1990, 1991; Lam *et al.*, 1999; Nerder *et al.*, 1999; Pinto *et al.*, 2001; Gazit-Rappaport *et al.*, 2003). Such asymmetries may be prevented by orthodontic therapy at an early stage in development. Because not all the orthodontic therapies show a positive result on masticatory function, the demonstration of the recovery of the altered muscular activation is important in order to know if the objective of the early treatment of the unilateral posterior crossbite was reached. This can be readily and routinely determined, during or after therapy, using electrognathography routinely to check, once again, the balance and coordination between sides. The possibility of checking the coordination of masticatory function would be an important achievement in improving our knowledge of function and motor control and changing our diagnostic and therapeutical approach to orthodontic therapy. The future of orthodontics cannot continue in a merely technical direction, but should evolve from a medical point of view, as the cranial growth and function of the stomatognathic system is one of the most complex issues in the medical field.

4.4.4.2.1 *Does unilateral posterior crossbite have any effect on posture?* (Figure 4.27)

"Posture" is currently a topic of huge interest, but reliable studies and tools suitable for evaluating them in an objective and scientific manner are still limited. This is due not only to technological constraints but also to the fact that postural behavior of the soma is easily influenced by many factors. As research stands currently, the results on the correlation between occlusion and pos-ture are in disagreement, as approximately 50% showed positive correlations whilst the other 50% displayed negative relationships.

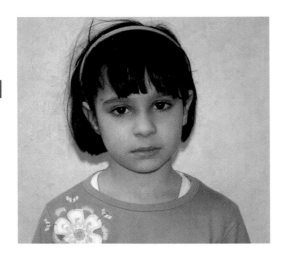
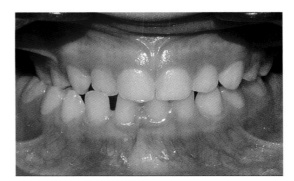

Figure 4.27 Face and occlusion of a child aged 6 years and 4 months with right posterior crossbite.

For the study of posture we are following the same research process as that carried out for mastication. We will not expand here on the topic as it is too complex in this context. The deep involvement of neuromuscular control during chewing in crossbite malocclusion strongly suggests a possible effect on body posture, and there are also the correlations between the masticatory muscles and the neck muscles during chewing to take into account (Eriksson *et al.*, 2000; Häggman-Henrikson and Eriksson, 2004; Häggman-Henrikson *et al.*, 2013). Again, to understand the phenomena we need to take a physiological approach. Hopefully, this will be the subject of a publication in the near future.

4.5 Anterior crossbite=neuromuscular syndrome (Figures 4.28 and 4.29)

Anterior crossbite can be defined as a malocclusion featuring *lingual occlusion of the upper anterior teeth* (incisors and canines) *with the lower anterior mandibular teeth*. The dental classification was described at the beginning of this chapter.

The functional aspect of this malocclusion is significantly different from that of unilateral posterior crossbite. We recall that the anterior teeth show a role of "sensory control" and guidance of the mandible in space, as well as protecting the diatoric contacts thanks to the laterotrusive and protrusive gliding function. The anterior region may be considered a true sense organ (Slavicek, 2002), very different from the posterior one that is dedicated to chewing.

Also, with unilateral anterior crossbite, it is important to consider not only the dental classification but also basal characteristics, which presents apparently similar features to unilateral posterior crossbite although on the sagittal plane as opposed to the frontal plane. It differs, therefore, in the *different impact it has on growth, which in this case regards the sagittal plane*.

Pathology of mastication

Unilateral anterior crossbite =
neuromuscular syndrome

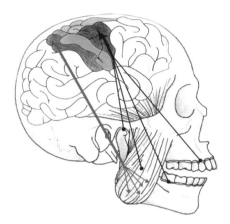

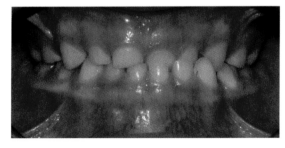 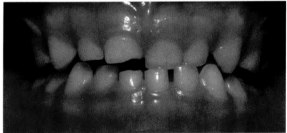

It is of clinical relevance, for successful orthodontic treatment, to consider not only the repositioning of teeth within the dental arches, but also, and above all, the effects of therapy on function.

Figure 4.28　Unilateral anterior crossbite=neuromuscular syndrome.

4.5.1　Effects of anterior crossbite on masticatory function

(Figures 4.30 and 4.31)

Taking into consideration the occlusal characteristics of unilateral anterior crossbite, the question was posed as to whether this type of malocclusion could display the same alterations to masticatory function or whether (taking into account the different functional role of the teeth involved) it could present different functional characteristics.

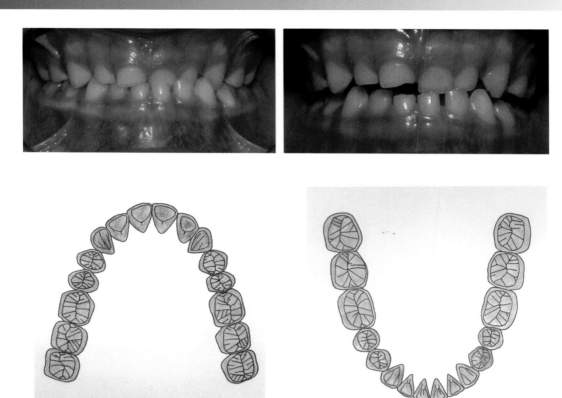

Figure 4.29 The functional aspects of anterior crossbite are different from that of posterior crossbite. The anterior region of the occlusion has a role of guidance of the mandible in the space, while the posterior regions are dedicated to support and mastication. *Source:* Redrawn from Slavicek (2002). Reproduced with permission from R. Slavicek.

This comparative study between mastication in unilateral anterior crossbite and unilateral posterior crossbite conditions was set up on the basis of reverse-sequence chewing cycle frequency. The results showed that the prevalence of reverse-sequence chewing cycles in anterior crossbite (without the involvement of any posterior premolar and/or molar teeth) was approximately 8–9% on the crossbite side and approximately 7–13% on the healthy side. Conversely, the percentage of reverse-sequence chewing cycles in the unilateral posterior crossbite patients proved (thus confirming previous results) significantly higher than the healthy side or the anterior crossbite side, showing a prevalence of 59% with soft bolus and 72% with hard bolus. The analysis of data concerning masticatory pattern features in patients with unilateral posterior crossbite confirmed the significant prevalence ($P < 0.001$) of reverse-sequence chewing cycles on the crossbite side as opposed to the healthy side, be it with soft or hard bolus types. The study revealed that in patients with unilateral anterior crossbite there was no significant number of reverse-sequence chewing cycles on the crossbite side as opposed to the healthy side, be it with a soft or hard bolus (Piancino *et al.*, 2012).

Unilateral anterior crossbite

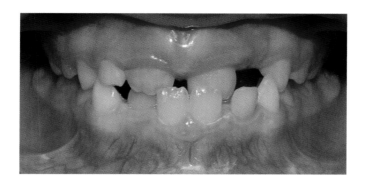

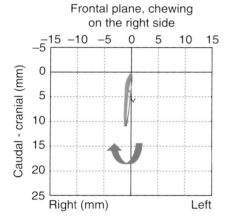

Frontal plane, chewing
on the right side

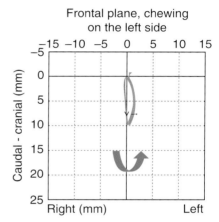

Frontal plane, chewing
on the left side

Figure 4.30   Chewing patterns of a patient with anterior crossbite. The closure direction is not altered on both sides. Green tracings: opening; red tracings: closing.

Furthermore, comparing patients with unilateral anterior crossbite and patients with unilateral posterior crossbite, the following was observed:

- On the non-crossbite side, there was no difference in the number of reverse-sequence chewing cycles between the posterior and anterior crossbite, whether with a soft or hard bolus.
- On the crossbite side, there was a significant higher number of reverse-sequence chewing cycles in posterior as opposed to anterior crossbite ($P < 0.01$), whether with a soft or hard bolus.
- Between the two sides, there was no difference in the anterior crossbites.
- Between the two sides, there was a difference in posterior crossbites.

It appears, then, that the percentage of reverse-sequence cycles recorded in unilateral anterior crossbite is low and that reverse-sequence cycles are present in significant numbers during chewing on the posterior crossbite side only. Thus, the functional asymmetry typical of unilateral posterior crossbite is not present in the anterior unilateral crossbite.

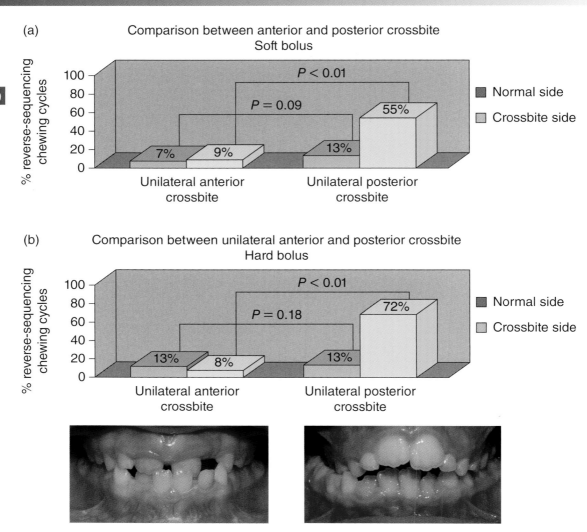

Figure 4.31 Comparison of the prevalence of reverse chewing cycles between unilateral anterior and posterior crossbites. There is no difference, during chewing, between sides in anterior crossbites, whereas there is significant difference between sides in unilateral posterior crossbites. Moreover, there is no difference between the normal sides of anterior versus posterior crossbites, whereas there is a significant difference between the anterior versus posterior crossbite side. *Source:* Piancino *et al.* (2012). Reproduced with permission from Oxford University Press.

These results show that the same type of malocclusion (i.e., crossbite) may register significantly different effects on masticatory function according to the dental region involved. In fact, when the malocclusion affects the dental area dedicated to the mandibular control in space (frontal-canine guidance) rather than bolus grinding, the reverse direction of closure in the masticatory cycle on the frontal plane would not have any functional reason (Piancino *et al.*, 2012). As well as unilateral anterior and posterior crossbite, there are also some mixed condition crossbites that involve both the anterior and posterior areas. In such cases, the dominant masticatory function is that of unilateral posterior crossbite.

In the light of the data gathered, we can conclude that the effect of the malocclusion on masticatory function depends on the functional role of teeth involved in the malocclusion, and that the effects *of anterior teeth on the chewing cycle in the frontal plane are significantly different from those of posterior teeth*.

References

Ahlgren J. (1967) Pattern of chewing and malocclusion of teeth. A clinical study. *Acta Odontol Scand* 25(1), 3–13.

Andrade AS, Gaviao MB, Gameiro GH, De Rossi M (2010) Characteristics of masticatory muscles in children with unilateral posterior crossbite. *Braz Oral Res* 24(2), 204–210.

Ben-Bassat Y, Yaffe A, Brin I, *et al.* (1993) Functional and morphological occlusal aspects in children treated for unilateral posterior cross-bite. *Eur J Orthod* 15, 57–63.

Bjork A, Krebs A, Solow B. (1964) A method for epidemiologic registration of malocclusion. *Acta Odontol Scand* 22(1), 27–41.

Bracco P, Solinas GF. (1979) Impiego e controllo della "placca funzionale bite" nel trattamento precoce del morso incrociato. *Mondo Ortodontico* 4, 1–11.

Bracco P, Piancino MG, Talpone F. (2002) Unilateral crossbite: electromyographic evidence of loss of masticatory muscle coordination during mastication. *Eur J Orthod* 4, 537 (abstract).

Brin I, Ben Bassat Y, Blustein Y, *et al.* (1996) Skeletal and functional effects of treatment for unilateral posterior crossbite. *Am J Orthod Dentofacial Orthop* 109, 173–179.

Cutroneo G, Piancino MG, Ramieri G, *et al.* (2012) Expression of muscle-specific integrins in masseter muscle fibers during malocclusion disease. *Int J Mol Med* 30(2), 235–242.

Da Silva Filho OG, Santamaria M Jr, Capelozza Filho L. (2007) Epidemiology of posterior crossbite in primary dentition. *J Clin Pediatr Dent* 32(1), 73–78.

Daskalogiannakis J. (2002) *Glossary of orthodontic terms*. Quintessence, Berlin.

Egermark-Eriksson I, Carlsson GE, Magnusson T, Thilander B. (1990) A longitudinal study of malocclusion in relation to signs and symptoms of craniomandibular disorders in children and adolescents. *Eur J Orthod* 12(4), 399–407.

Engström C, Kiliaridis S, Thilander B. (1986) The relationship between masticatory function and craniofacial morphology. II. A histological study in the growing rat fed a soft diet. *Eur J Orthod* 8(4), 271–279.

Enlow D. (1986) *Handbook of facial growth*. WB Saunders, Philadelphia, PA.

Eriksson PO, Häggman-Henrikson B, Nordh E, Zafar H. (2000) Co-ordinated mandibular and head–neck movements during rhythmic jaw activities in man. *J Dent Res* 79(6), 1378–1384.

Frongia G, Bracco P, Piancino MG. (2013) Three-dimensional cephalometry: a method for the identification and for the orientation of the skull after cone beam-computed tomographic scan. *J Craniofac Surg* 24(3), e308–e311.

Favaloro A, Speranza G, Rezza S, *et al.* (2009) Muscle-specific integrins in masseter muscle fibers of chimpanzees: an immunohistochemical study. *Folia Histochem Cytobiol* 47(4), 551–558.

Gazit-Rappaport T, Weinreb M, Gazit E. (2003) Quantitative evaluation of lip symmetry in functional asymmetry. *Eur J Orthod* 25, 443–450.

Häggman-Henrikson B, Eriksson PO. (2004) Head movements during chewing: relation to size and texture of bolus. *J Dent Res* 83(11), 864–868.

Häggman-Henrikson B, Nordh E, Eriksson PO. (2013) Increased sternocleidomastoid, but not trapezius, muscle activity in response to increased chewing load. *Eur J Oral Sci* 121(5), 443–449.

Harrison JE, Ashby D. (2003) Orthodontic treatment for posterior crossbites. *Cochrane Syst Rev* (2), CD000979.

Hinton RJ. (1981) Changes in articular eminence morphology with dental function. *Am J Phys Anthropol* 54(4), 439–455.

Ishii N, Soma K, Toda K. (2002) Response properties of periodontal mechanoreceptors in rats, in vitro. *Brain Res Bull* 58, 357–361.

Johnsen S, Trulsson M. (2003) Receptive field properties of human periodontal afferents responding to loading of premolar and molar teeth. *J Neurophysiol* 89, 1478–1487.

Katoh M, Taira M, Katakura N, Nakamura Y. (1982) Cortically induced effects on trigeminal motoneurons after transection of the brainstem at the pontobulbar junction in the cat. *Neurosci Lett* 33, 141–146.

Kiliaridis S, Thilander B, Kjellberg H, *et al.* (1999) Effect of low masticatory function on condylar growth: a morphometric study in the rat. *Am J Orthod Dentofacial Orthop* 116(2), 121–125.

Kiliaridis S, Mahboubi PH, Raadsheer MC, Katsaros C. (2007) Ultrasonographic thickness of the masseter muscles in growing individuals with unilateral crossbite. *Angle Orthod* 77(4), 607–611.

Lam PH, Sadowsky C, Omerza F. (1999) Mandibular asymmetry and condylar position in children with unilateral posterior crossbite. *Am J Orthod Dentofacial Orthop* 115, 569–575.

Lewin A. (1985) *Electrognathographics: atlas of diagnostic procedures and interpretation.* Quintessence, Berlin.

Lund JP, Kolta A. (2006) Generation of the central masticatory pattern and its modification by sensory feedback. *Dysphagia* 21(3), 167–174.

Lund JP, Scott G, Kolta A, Westberg GR. (1999) Role of cortical inputs and brainstem interneuron populations in patterning mastication. In: *Neurobiology of mastication. From molecular to system approach* (eds Y Nakamura, GJ Sessle). Elsevier Science, Tokyo, pp. 504–514.

Lundeen HC, Gibbs CH. (1982) *Advances in occlusion.* J Wright–PSG, Boston, MA.

Martín C, Alarcón JA, Palma JC. (2000) Kinesiographic study of the mandible in young patients with unilateral posterior crossbite. *Am J Orthod Dentofacial Orthop* 118(5), 541–548.

Martín C, Palma JC, Alamán JM, *et al.* (2012) Longitudinal evaluation of sEMG of masticatory muscles and kinematics of mandible changes in children treated for unilateral cross-bite. *J Electromyogr Kinesiol* 22(4), 620–628.

Moller E, Troelstrup B. (1975) Functional and morphologic asymmetry in children with unilateral cross-bite. *J Dent Res* 5(Special issue), 178.

Morquette P, Lavoie R, Fhima MD, *et al.* (2012) Generation of the masticatory central pattern and its modulation by sensory feedback. *Prog Neurobiol* 96(3), 340–355.

Neff P. (1999) *TMJ occlusion and function.* http://peterneffdds.com/blog, http://www.amazon.com/TMJ-occlusion-function-Peter-Neff/dp/B0006RE5SK (accessed October 2, 2015).

Nerder PH, Bakke M, Solow B. (1999) The functional shift of the mandible in unilateral posterior crossbite and the adaptation of the temporomandibular joints: a pilot study. *Eur J Orthod* 21, 155–166.

Onozuka M, Fujita M, Watanabe K, *et al.* (2002) Mapping brain region activity during chewing: a functional magnetic resonance imaging study. *J Dent Res* 81, 743–746.

Piancino MG, Talpone F, Rampa C, *et al.* (2006a) Epidemiological study of crossbites – classification and postero-anterior cephalometric evaluation. *Eur J Orthod* 28(6), e249.

Piancino MG, Talpone F, Dalmasso P, *et al.* (2006b) Reverse-sequencing chewing patterns before and after treatment of children with a unilateral posterior crossbite. *Eur J Orthod* 28(5), 480–484.

Piancino MG, Farina D, Talpone F, *et al.* (2009) Muscular activation during reverse and non-reverse chewing cycles in unilateral posterior crossbite. *Eur J Oral Sci* 117(2), 122–128.

Piancino MG, Comino E, Talpone F, *et al.* (2012) Reverse-sequencing chewing patterns evaluation in anterior versus posterior unilateral crossbite patients. *Eur J Orthod* 34(5), 536–541.

Piancino MG, Cannavale R, Dalmasso P, *et al.* (2015a) Condylar asymmetry in patients with juvenile idiopathic arthritis: could it be a sign of a possible temporomandibular joints involvement? *Semin Arthritis Rheum* 42(2), 208–213.

Piancino MG, Falla D, Merlo A, *et al.* (2015) Masseter activation, during chewing, in unilateral posterior crossbite before/after therapy. Abstract, IADR General Session, Boston, MA, March 11–14.

Pinto AS, Buschang PH, Throckmorton GS, Chen P. (2001) Morphological and positional asymmetries of young children with functional unilateral posterior crossbite. *Am J Orthodod Dentofacial Orthop* 120, 513–520.

Pirttiniemi P, Kantomaa T, Lahtela P. (1990) Relationship between craniofacial and condyle path asymmetry in unilateral cross-bite patients. *Eur J Orthod* 12, 408–413.

Pirttiniemi P, Raustia A, Kantomaa T, Pyhtinen J (1991) Relationships of bicondylar position to occlusal asymmetry. *Eur J Orthod* 13, 441–445.

Poikela A, Kantomaa T, Pirttiniemi P. (1997) Craniofacial growth after a period of unilateral masticatory function in young rabbits. *Eur J Oral Sci* 105(4), 331–337.

Purves D, Augustine GJ, Fitzpatrick, *et al.* (2000) *Neuroscienze* (trans. RLucchi, APoli, MVirgili). Zanichelli, Bologna.

Saitoh I, Yamada C, Hayasaki H, *et al.* (2010) Is the reverse cycle during chewing abnormal in children with primary dentition. *J Oral Rehabil* 37(1), 26–33.

Santana-Mora U, Lopez Cedrun J, Mora MJ, *et al.* (2013). Temporomandibular disorders: the habitual chewing side syndrome. *PLoS One* 8(4), e59980.

Sever E, Marion L, Ovsenik M. (2011) Relationship between masticatory cycle morphology and unilateral crossbite in the primary dentition. *Eur J Orthod* 33, 620–627.

Slavicek R. (2002) *The masticatory organ: functions and dysfunctions*. Gamma Medizinisch-wissenschaftliche Fortbildung-AG, Klosterneuburg.

Sonnesen L, Bakke M, Solow B. (2001) Bite force in pre-orthodontic children with unilateral crossbite. *Eur J Orthod* 23(6), 741–749.

Thilander B. (1995) Basic mechanisms in craniofacial growth. *Acta Odontol Scand* 53(3), 144–151.

Thilander B, Lennartsson B. (2002) A study of children with unilateral posterior crossbite, treated and untreated, in the deciduous dentition – occlusal and skeletal characteristics of significance in predicting the long-term outcome. *J Orofac Orthop* 63(5), 371–383.

Thilander B, Bjerklin K (2012) Posterior crossbite and temporomandibular disorders: need for orthodontic treatment. *Eur J Orthod* 34(6), 667–673.

Thilander B, Carlsson GE, Ingervall B. (1976) Postnatal development of the human temporomandibular joint. I. A histological study. *Acta Odontol Scand* 34(2), 117–126.

Thilander B, Wahlund S, Lennartsson B. (1984) The effect of early interceptive treatment in children with posterior cross-bite. *Eur J Orthod* 6(1), 25–34.

Throckmorton GS, Buschang PH, Hayasaki H, Pinto AS. (2001) Changes in the masticatory cycle following treatment of posterior unilateral crossbite in children. *Am J Orthod Dentofacial Orthop* 120, 521–529.

Wilding RJ, Lewin A. (1994) The determination of optimal human jaw movements based on their association with chewing performance. *Arch Oral Biol* 39(4), 333–343.

Yoshino K, Kawagishi S, Takatsuki Y, Amano N. (1999) Different roles of the primary motor and ventral premotor cortex in jaw movements. In: *Neurobiology of mastication. From molecular to system approach* (eds YNakamura, GJSessle). Elsevier Science, Tokyo, pp. 515–517.

Chapter 5

Therapy with Function Generating Bite Appliance: Actions and Effects on Malocclusion and Masticatory Function

Contents

Understanding Masticatory Function in Unilateral Crossbites, First Edition. Maria Grazia Piancino and Stephanos Kyrkanides.
© 2016 John Wiley & Sons, Inc. Published 2016 by John Wiley & Sons, Inc.

5.1 Orthognathodontic therapy aimed to restore physiological neuromuscular equilibrium to the stomatognathic system

As described in Chapter 4, unilateral posterior crossbite is a malocclusion characterized by worsening structural and functional asymmetry to such an extent that *this form of crossbite may be considered as much more than a simple malocclusion*. Awareness of the complexity of this pathology is a vital factor in recognizing the signs and symptoms that patients display, in order to choose the most appropriate therapy to treat all the areas involved, through teeth. *Correction of functional asymmetry in its early stages of development* allows restoration of function and

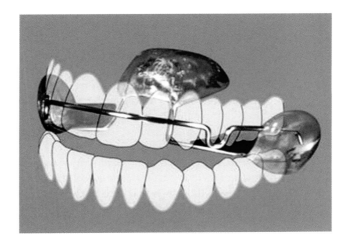

Figure 5.1 FGB appliance with posterior bite planes. *Source:* Courtesy of P. Bracco, Piancino *et al.* (2006). Reproduced with permission from Oxford University Press.

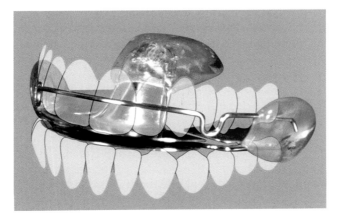

Figure 5.2 FGB appliance with double anterior and posterior bite planes. *Source:* Courtesy of P. Bracco, Castroflorio *et al.* (2004). Reproduced with permission from John Wiley & Sons.

harmonious growth of the stomatognathic system; but to achieve this goal, *non-traumatic therapies that respect the biological and physiological wellbeing of the structures* are needed (Deshayes, 2006; Gorbonos *et al.*, 2013; Simoes, 2013).

Research shows that functional asymmetry (and its resulting effects on growth) can be corrected with prompt use of an orthognathodontic functionalizing appliance called function generating bite (FGB) (Figures 5.1, 5.2). This device works, via the teeth, to restore function and *correct dental malocclusion*. The gerund term "function generating" underlines the continuous, rhythmic action of the appliance. The aim is to create correct masticatory function through the use of metal bite planes that act as elective therapeutic structures of the functionalizing appliance. Thus, any therapeutic tool used by the orthodontist must *respect the principles of gnathology*; that is, of physiological masticatory function. The orthodontic appliances currently available (both fixed and removable) successfully correct dental issues, but scientific proof of the restoration of masticatory function is still not considered.

Research into mastication shows that the fact that restoration of function after a malocclusion is corrected with an FGB appliance is not a coincidence, and that it is worth exploring further the features of the appliance in order to understand the reasons and clinical importance of these results. This chapter, which provides an explanation of the actions and effects of functional appliances that simultaneously correct the dental issue and restore masticatory function, is an important step in the research into chewing cycles. Clinicians may immediately see a physiological improvement in all developing structures of young children thanks to orthognathodontic intervention with the FGB appliance. We are sure that, with a little effort, it will be easy to understand how this functional therapy can improve not only dental conditions, but also, and above all, the subsequent growth (Moss and Salentijn 1969a,b; Enlow and Bang, 1965; Duterloo and Enlow, 1970; Enlow, 1990) and health of young children's stomatognathic systems, *avoiding any side effects* that may threaten function. The ideal aim of any orthodontic treatment is to reposition teeth and support bones in a position of maximum equilibrium from a structural and neuromuscular point of view, avoiding cusp-to-cusp contacts in order *to achieve a balanced stomatognathic system that is constantly stable, without the need for any form of compensation.* When this is not possible or when traumatic therapies are adopted that do not respect biological and physiological wellbeing, the appliance exerts pressure on teeth, creating *premature contacts that lead to deviation of the mandible, dislocation of the condyle, and neuromuscular and functional imbalance* (Figure 5.3). The FGB appliance allows the repositioning of teeth whilst fully respecting the physiological condition of the TMJ and avoiding harmful misaligned dental contacts.

To understand how and why the functionalizing device corrects not only teeth but also function, we must study the device's features. First of all, we would like to point out that the first scientific articles on functional devices date back to Bracco and Solinas (1979a, b), and that the actions and effects of this type of device have been studied and refined over a long period of time. The first example of such a device with an anterior bite plane was created in 1969–1970 by Professor A. J. Cervera, a Spanish pediatrician, to whom we can attribute the first use of a *resilient metal bite, smooth and free-moving in the oral cavity with the objective of leveling out the occlusal plane and rebalancing the function of the frontal-canine guide.* Following this, we can thank Professor P. Bracco for having understood the *gnathological potential* of this device, and then continuing the research work and adapting it (using the same principles) to various cranial typologies. This was achieved thanks to his challenging work and to the gnathologic concepts he had the opportunity to learn from the most important gnathologists in the world as described in the preface. On this basis, he very soon understood the importance of correcting the crossbite malocclusion. In fact, the FGB appliance was manufactured for the correction of crossbite, as we shall soon see. I am proud to write his own definition of the FGB appliance: FGB is *"a revolutionary functionalizing orthognathodontic device* because it allows spontaneous repositioning of the mandible in a centered position during its use and during orthodontic movement" (Bracco and Piancino, 2009).

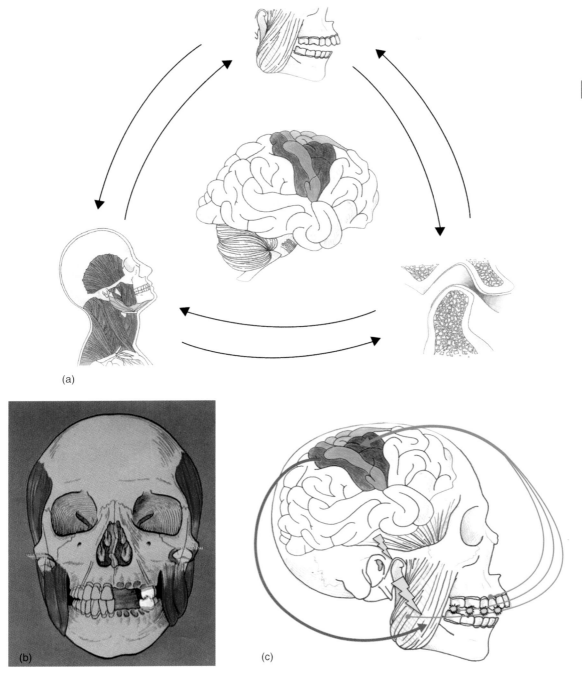

Figure 5.3 (a) The stomatognathic system. Relationships between dental occlusion, TMJ, and neuromuscular control. (b, c) Premature contacts cause deviation of the mandible, dislocation of the condyle, and muscular imbalance in the three planes of space. *Source for the muscles:* Neff (1999). *Source for the brain:* Purves *et al.* (2000). Reproduced with the permission of Sinauer Associates.

148

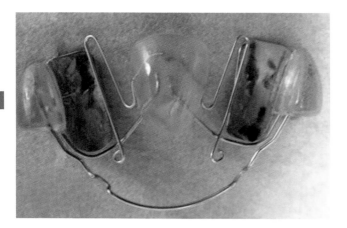

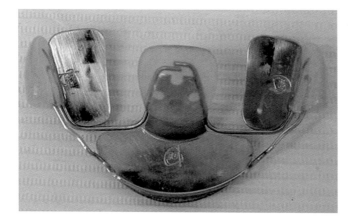

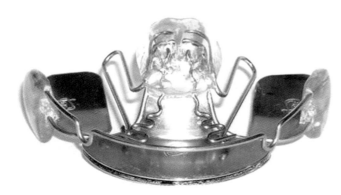

Figure 5.4 FGB appliance with posterior bite planes (*top*), with anterior and posterior bite planes (*middle*), and with double anterior and posterior bite planes (*bottom*).

The FGB appliance is a functionalizing device, individually wrapped, made of acrylic resin and characterized by posterior metal bites in resilient steel. We can unquestionably define it as a gnathological device. This claim is supported by an explanation of the dental–alveolar–basal actions and effects of the appliance, but, as already mentioned, in order to reason in gnathological terms (i.e. terms of masticatory function) and to *"cure" the functional alterations of the stomatognathic system via the teeth*, we should first act according to physiological and biological principles. In other words, we need to put aside localized or mechanical reasoning based purely or principally on teeth and *learn to view teeth as an integral part of a complex functional system*; that is, the stomatognathic system. The role of teeth in the stomatognathic system is anything but secondary. They are dominant structures and we have explained in depth how sensory data arriving from the teeth influence the neuromuscular programming of the mandibular position. According to what we know on this topic today, we *cannot consider moving teeth mechanically without worrying about functional consequences and the future health of the stomatognathic system in young and old patients*. The human masticatory system is a "multifunctional" organ dedicated not only to mastication but also to deglutition, speech, and head and body posture; *it contributes to the mental and physical wellbeing of patients* (Slavicek, 2002). In other words, *the good health of the stomatognathic system influences the quality of life in our patients and all of us*. Thus, it is worth applying gnathological concepts to orthognathodontic therapies in order to achieve these highly important results.

Functionalizing appliances are (Figure 5.4):

- appliances with two posterior bite plates;
- appliances with an anterior bite plate and two posterior bite plates;
- appliances with a double anterior bite plate and two posterior bite plates.

Note that the posterior bite plates are always present, in all models. Following clinical research, these bites became a structural part of the devices. This book looks at appliances with two posterior bite plates, namely *FGB appliance*s, as these are the ones most commonly adopted for correction of unilateral posterior crossbite.

5.2 Dental–alveolar–basal actions and effects of function generating bite appliances

A thorough comprehension of dental–alveolar–basal actions and effects is important in order to understand the gnathological features of these functionalizing devices and their action (via teeth) on skeletal structures, as well as the vectoriality and type of orthodontic forces that influence bone growth/development. Functionalizing devices are different from other appliances in two main aspects:

1. the self-regulation of mandibular position in space and the self-regulation of orthodontic forces;
2. the simultaneous performance of actions in the three planes of space and in different sectors (skeletal, dental, and muscular).

This makes the FGB unique in its field, not only from an orthodontic point of view, but also from a gnathological point of view. The simultaneous performance of actions and the self-adjustment of the mandible are original features that oblige us to rethink our usual ideas. These features differ greatly from traditional mechanics where actions are sector based and never unitary, as well as pre-established and never self-regulating, with the final objective being dental repositioning without any or very little consideration of function, functional compensation, or neuromuscular equilibrium.

The general actions and effects of the FGB can be summarized as in the following list, which outlines the more detailed topics undertaken in this chapter:

- disengagement and self-repositioning of the mandible;
- leveling and alignment of the occlusal plane, avoiding trauma and protecting dental cuspids;
- muscle anchorage;
- possibility of symmetric and asymmetric activation;
- dental repositioning with self-regulating, intermittent forces;
- re-education of the tongue, stabilization of the device;
- progressive reprogramming of neural motor control via self-regulation.

5.2.1 Characteristics of the appliance components

The main parts of the FGB appliance work together simultaneously during swallowing and phonation, both of which activate the appliance; each component has its own precise functional role.

The FGB appliance (Figure 5.5) is composed of:

- resilient stainless steel bite plates;
- buccal shields;
- expansion springs;
- palatal button.

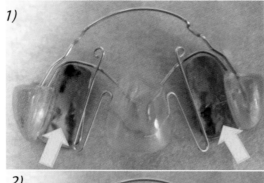

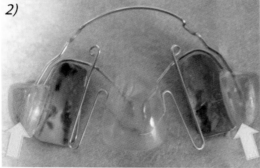

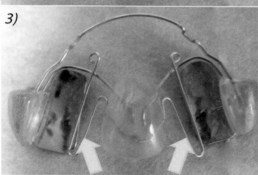

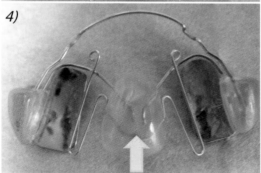

Figure 5.5 FGB appliance components: (1) resilient stainless steel bite planes, (2) buccal shields, (3) expansion springs, (4) palatal button.

We will now look at these individual elements of the appliance, describing the actions and effects of each component. Even though the elements will be described one by one, all the actions and effects of the components are simultaneous. In general, an FGB appliance is characterized by self-regulating activation, progressive reprogramming of neural motor control, restoral of the reverse chewing pattern and relative muscular balance, and improvement of symmetry of function and growth. For this reason, it has important actions and effects on the cranial–maxillofacial structures that will be expressly described.

But the following particular characteristics, which will be explained in Sections 5.3 and 5.4, are important as well:

- non-cariogenic;
- no need for any change of the appliance in the event of emergence of a permanent tooth, and easily adapted in the event of ectopic eruption of a permanent tooth;
- once the malocclusion has been treated, it can be used for "active retention" as it adapts constantly to growing structures, not only neutralizing the risk of relapse, but continuously stimulating growth and balancing;
- never restrictive;
- minimum time necessary at the dental chair, allowing excellent organization of work time.

5.2.1.1 Resilient stainless steel bite planes (Figure 5.6)

Actions and effects:

1. Disengagement and self-repositioning of the mandible in a centered position for improvement of joint functional movement.
2. Occlusal plane leveling and alignment of the dental arches, avoiding trauma and protecting dental cusps.
3. Contribution to the orthodontic repositioning of the teeth.

The resilient stainless steel bite plates free to move in the mouth are an essential element of the FGB appliance and represent the principal difference between this and other orthodontic appliances. No other removable or functional appliance (either currently in use or described in the literature)

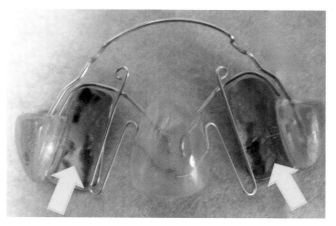

Figure 5.6 FGB appliance component: resilient stainless steel bite planes.

has this same feature. Many appliances have occlusal components inserted between the arches, but none of these feature a resilient metal bite plate that is smooth and free-moving in the oral cavity in order to level and balance the occlusal plane.

The posterior metal bite plates have evolved from a research path involving both construction issues and clinical application in thousands of cases. They were designed and fine-tuned following the initial device concept of A. J. Cervera (featuring only the anterior metal bite plate). This appliance aimed to supply homogeneous leveling of the frontal sector and to restore the fronto-canine guide in hypodivergent patients with dental deep bite. However, in the 1970s there was no functional device in existence to correct the opposite malocclusion; i.e. dental anterior open bite in hyperdivergent patients. Having understood well that crossbite can be linked with dental anterior open bite and that the correction of this dual functional malocclusion in hyperdivergent patients is extremely complex, P. Bracco decided (Figure 5.7)

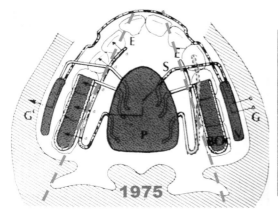
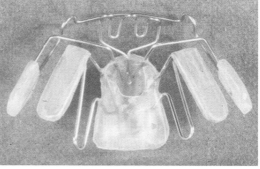

Figure 5.7 Old version of FGB appliance with resin bite planes (drawing and prototype). G: cheek; E: expansion springs; S: structural wire; P: palatal button; BO: occlusal plate (resin); V: buccal shield; d: dental point contact. *Source:* P. Bracco, Turin, Italy. Reproduced with permission from P. Bracco.

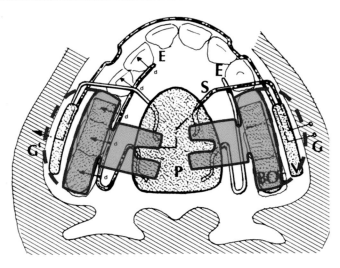

Figure 5.8 Old version of FGB appliance with the anterior metallic bite plane used in the posterior region. *Source:* P. Bracco, Turin, Italy. Reproduced with permission from P. Bracco.

to use the same gnathological principle of anterior metal bite plates for the posterior molar and premolar areas. Erring on the side of caution, at the beginning, posterior bite plates in resin were used as this was the material used at that time for removable appliances (Figure 5.7). After 4 or 5 years, it emerged that this material was not ideal, it became clear that the functional forces were indenting the resin, limiting freedom of movement (especially laterally), and that this led to it being chipped or smashed. The results were unsuccessful because of this indented resin, which imprisoned the mandible instead of releasing it. Moreover, the resin plates exploded. Thus, it was decided to produce some posterior metal bite plates in stainless steel, adapting the anterior bite plates (the only ones known at that time) modeled for bespoke purposes and anchored to the palatal button (Figure 5.8). The downside was that the tongue rubbed against the metallic edges of the palatal side, causing pain. To solve this problem, it was decided to anchor the metal bite plates to the buccal shields, but the first attempts were still unsuccessful as the resin was too easily broken.

This alteration called for in-depth studies of mechanical physics applied to dental technology in order to eliminate contrasting actions and effects. Here, we will not linger on the various laboratory experiments carried out, but we would like to underline that the research process was neither simple nor quick – numerous attempts were made to refine the necessary materials and laboratory techniques. It immediately emerged that there was *an advantage in achieving bite plates that did not indent like resin but "cupped" with dental pressure, thanks to the flexibility of a resilient stainless steel, thus allowing the action of self-repositioning of the mandible in all stages of orthognathodontic treatment.* It was at this point that the FGB appliance was renamed, from "functional" to "functionalizing."

5.2.1.1.1 Disengagement and self-repositioning of the mandible in a centered position for improvement of joint functional movement

One of the most important actions of the bite plates is that of *disengaging the mandible from occlusion.* This is carried out with the FGB appliance thanks to the elasticity and fluid movement of the metallic bites, which allow the mandible to find its ideal structural and

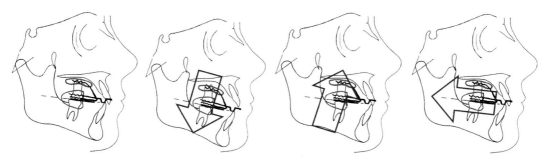

Figure 5.9   Disengagement of the mandible and self-repositioning with FGB appliance during swallowing. *Source:* P. Bracco, Turin, Italy. Reproduced with permission from P. Bracco.

neuromuscular equilibrium at any stage of the therapy. In this way, the mandible is no longer influenced by intercuspal contacts that force it into a defined position pushing the stomatognathic system to produce neuromuscular compensation. Instead, it is free to self-reposition in the three spatial planes on the basis of individual structural characteristics (Figure 5.9). This is plainly visible in children with unilateral posterior crossbite – as soon as they are fitted with the FGB appliance, without any activation, the mandible moves into a central position that the malocclusion (in maximum intercuspation) does not allow. At this point it is useful to remember that the possibility of self-repositioning of the mandible during the age of development and up to the initial stages of treatment, along with functional rebalancing, is important for harmonious development of skeletal structures in children (Figure 5.10). The TMJ is particularly sensitive to compensation and adjustment, and it is fundamental in the future functioning of the child's cephalic zone. In fact, we know that at birth this joint is still to be formed and that the postnatal change is huge. From histological studies by Thilander, we know that the TMJ is characterized by an adaptive type of growth (Figure 5.10) (Thilander *et al.*, 1976; Ingervall *et al.*, 1976; Engström *et al.*, 1986; Thilander and Bjerklin, 2012). This means that malocclusion and treatment have an influence on the TMJ development. Thus, all the means that we can use to improve function and physiology of this joint in the developmental phase are important for the child's structural and functional development. From this point of view, the FGB is extremely useful because it allows us to halt an imbalanced and asymmetric function with mandibular dislocation, in order to restore (from the very outset of therapy) the positional equilibrium of the mandible and its movement (self-regulating and not previously established), at any stage of treatment.

When the appliance is in place, the mandible performs correctly according to physiological standards – free from premature dental contacts, performing smooth condylar tracings, with positive effects on the trophism of all elements of the stomatognathic system. Thus, the adoption of an FGB appliance during the stage of growth allows the TMJ to grow supported by good dental and occlusal contacts and smooth movements. All action is aimed at *normalizing the system*, eliminating premature contacts and repositioning the mandible in a centered position, without causing any harmful effects.

The adaptive growth of the TMJ, which benefits from the balanced dental arches and occlusion produced by the support of the bite plate, together with the gnathological action of disengaging and self-repositioning (made possible by the smoothness of the material), shows us that the *use of a resilient steel bite is preferable to any other type of material*.

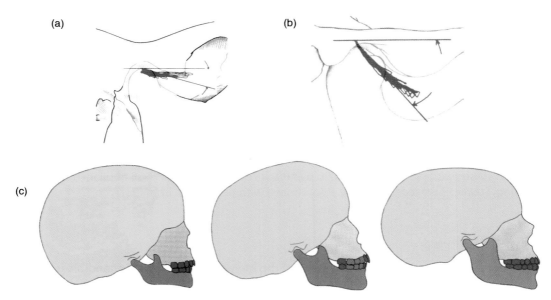

Figure 5.10 Adaptive growth of the TMJ during different developmental stages from deciduous dentition (a) to permanent dentition (b) (top). Functional balancing is important for harmonious growth of the joint and skeletal structures (c) (bottom). *Source for part (c):* Slavicek (2002). Reproduced with permission from R. Slavicek.

In order to carry out the physiological and self-repositioning actions described, the FGB appliance's bite includes the following features:

- *It is not attached to teeth* and does not restrict either the upper or lower teeth or the mandible in a fixed position. Instead, it "cups" the teeth and allows free movement of the mandible at all stages of therapy (from the beginning, both when the malocclusion is present and during the dental repositioning), allowing its self-repositioning.
- *It adapts* to dental pressure, thanks to its resilience.
- *It protects* dental cusps from premature contacts.
- *It levels* the occlusal plane and *simultaneously aligns* the upper and lower dental arches.
- *It allows* the transmission of a physiological *force* to teeth, which is intermittent, and not continuous nor enforced but self-regulated.

The "imprint" is the mark left by teeth on the bite device after use, both on the upper and lower part of the appliance (Figure 5.11). *This is due to simultaneous pressure of the teeth in both the upper and lower arches*, and this is a unique feature of the resilient steel bite. It is significant because even in the event of multiple imprints the mandible maintains freedom of movement, as the point of contact between the teeth and metal bite is always punctiform as opposed to molded (as occurs with resin). The traditional resin bite is "indented" during the early stages of therapy, obliging the mandible to return to the same initial position every time and preventing continuous repositioning as happens with an FGB appliance.

Furthermore, the "imprint" is a sign of the occlusal *force* imprinted simultaneously on the upper and lower dental arches, which leads to gradual leveling of the occlusal plane by means

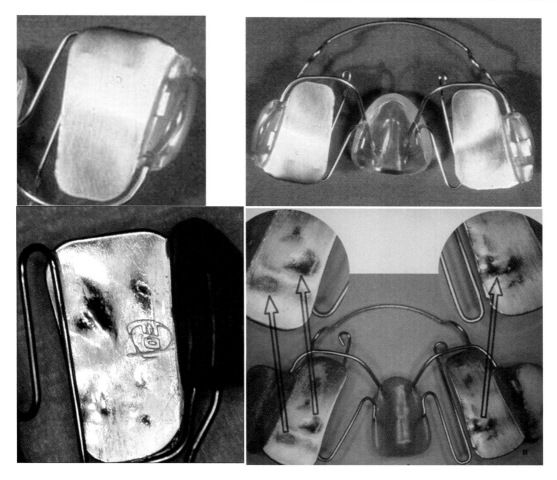

Figure 5.11   New, resilient stainless steel bites (*top*); bites after use with cupped signs (*bottom*).

of (intermittent and physiological forces, during swallowing) (Figure 5.12). We know that in the majority of cases malocclusions are due to problems of both upper and lower dental arches and bones, almost never of one alone. The FGB appliance corrects the malocclusion by aligning teeth in both arches in a balanced and self-regulating manner. This is the first essential step toward *normalization of the system with the elimination of premature contacts and the recentering of the mandible.*

Gradually, as restored equilibrium is achieved and the mandible acquires increased freedom of movement, the bites can display not only "imprint" signs, but also *"gothic arch-like traces" that represent the active, physiological, and rhythmic movement of the mandible.* This important type of mark indicates correct mandibular movement, free from teeth contacts, and *beneficial effects for the trophism* of the entire stomatognathic system.

The spontaneous induction of rhythmic and physiological movements is made possible by the muscular (not dental) anchoring and by the smooth and resilient surface of the bite plates; it is then logical that the FGB appliance, which does not restrict the dental arches at any point

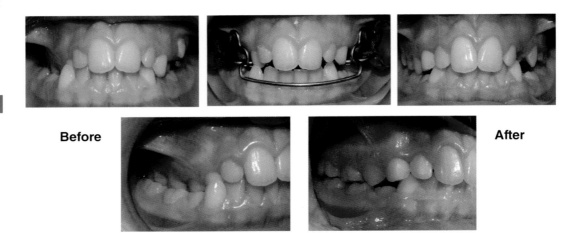

Before　　　　　　　　　　　　　　　　　　　　　　　**After**

Figure 5.12 Leveling of the occlusal plane before and after the use of FGB appliance in mixed dentition.

(whether upper or lower) and allows the disengagement of the mandible, may be considered *primarily a gnathological appliance*.

Regarding this issue, we must not forget that the use of a metal plate is common in gnathological recordings of the likes of Gerber recordings or axiography (Figure 5.13). This is because the metal plate permits the mandible the maximum freedom of movement possible and allows reliable recording of mandibular border movements, which can then be transferred to a stereographic recording in order to design prosthetic devices that respect physiological movement. At the same time, the therapeutic goal of the metal bite is to eliminate anomalous dental contacts that impede correct mandibular movement. *The functionalizing device is based on the same physiological rules used in reconstructive prosthetic technology, in full respect of masticatory function.* In this way, prosthodontists will treat orthodontic patients, when necessary, according to analogous and homogeneous rules.

Only a functionalizing and muscle anchoring appliance that does not imprison teeth or any other element of the structure and that is totally free of metal wires that affect occlusal contact can allow the automatic establishment of physiological movement (such as "gothic arch-like" traces) (Figure 5.14). This is one of the reasons why patients with TMJ disorders who are treated with functionalizing devices display significant improvement in post-therapy axiographic tracking (Piancino *et al.*, 2008).

Thus, the FGB appliance leads to improved function of the stomatognathic system, both together with orthodontic movement.

5.2.1.1.2 *Leveling of the occlusal plane and alignment of dental arches without the risk of trauma, whilst protecting dental cusps*

Another feature of metal bites is the leveling of the occlusal plane achieved whilst preventing premature cusp–cusp contacts, and with simultaneous action in the upper and lower arches. *Protection from premature contacts*, which are often an inevitable consequence during orthodontic movement of teeth, allows (at any stage of treatment) the physiological repositioning of the mandible. In fact, cusp-to-cusp contacts generate peripheral inputs that are transmitted to the central nervous system by mechanoreceptors; these peripheral inputs are

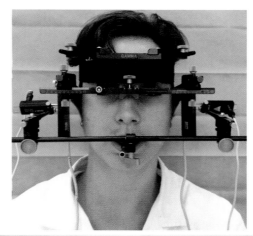

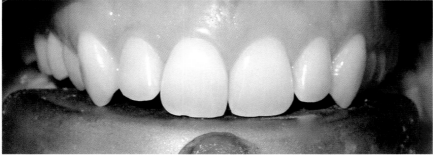

Figure 5.13   Axiography recording with metallic clutch.

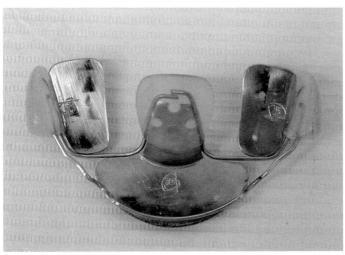

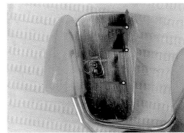

Figure 5.14   Signs on the bite planes after use of FGB appliance looking like "gothic arches."
Source: Courtesy of P. Bracco.

perceived as a sign of danger to the structures, and activate a neuromuscular program aimed at avoiding such contacts, which leads to mandibular displacement of varying levels of magnitude. Control of these inputs is thus important in order to allow a physiological reprogramming of motor control, a centered mandibular position, and *to avoid undesirable or iatrogenic mandibular shift*.

Furthermore, the bite action takes place simultaneously within the upper and lower arches, leveling the occlusal plane with self-regulating force. In the event of unilateral posterior crossbite, in the initial stages different forces are applied to the teeth in the crossbite area, where occlusal asymmetry and misalignment are of more importance, before gradually becoming uniform until the entire occlusal plane is leveled. As the dental repositioning takes place, the system is gradually regulated and forces are symmetrized (Figure 5.12).

Self-regulation of forces is an extremely important concept, yet, unfortunately, it is still relatively unknown. Huge amounts of effort, time, articles, and congresses have been dedicated to the "mechanics" of fixed devices, whilst often (almost always) forgetting the "bio" aspect of dental movement and the physiology of the stomatognathic system in favor of purely mechanical issues. The concept of "self-regulating forces" is one of the vital principles of the FGB appliance, which is activated by the masticatory muscles. We know that there is a large amount of peripheral data sent to the brain by the receptors of the stomatognathic system, in a quick and precise manner, and the brain response in terms of periodontal–masseteric reflex opening, and so on, takes place, via masticatory muscles, with just as much speed and precision; in fact, the motor endplates of this muscle control a few muscle fibers, permitting great precision of neuromuscular control. A child (or patient in general) has a neuromuscular system that controls not only the force levels that the tooth can tolerate, but also the activation times of the appliance. At the points of greatest misalignment, occlusal force will never be beyond the tolerance level of the patient's stomatognathic system. Neuromuscular control adjusts muscle contraction to the system and, as the more seriously misaligned teeth come into alignment, other teeth are involved also until physiological and non-traumatic alignment is achieved along the occlusal plane – this process is entirely unforced and needs no compensation by the mandible in space as unavoidably happens with fixed appliances.

As the FGB appliance works on three spatial planes, it is not possible to separate the action of occlusal leveling from that of dental alignment, both of which occur simultaneously.

5.2.1.1.3 Contribution to the orthodontic repositioning of the teeth
See Section 5.2.1.3 on expansion springs.

5.2.1.2 Buccal shields (Figure 5.15)
Actions and effects:

1. *Muscle anchorage* and rebalance of function.
2. Self-regulated *transmission of muscle force* to expansion springs.
3. Production of *symmetric and asymmetric forces*, without side-effects, to achieve forces coherent with the therapeutic goals.
4. Creation of *decompression spaces* for the formation of new bone tissue to provide dental stability.
5. Anchorage of the arches and optionals.

5.2.1.2.1 Muscle anchorage and reequilibrium of function
Buccal shields (like bites) are a special feature of the FGB appliance and deserve separate discussion. These shields provide the FGB's muscle anchorage. In fact, the FGB is characterized by exclusively punctiform contacts *without any form of dental anchorage* and, when the mouth

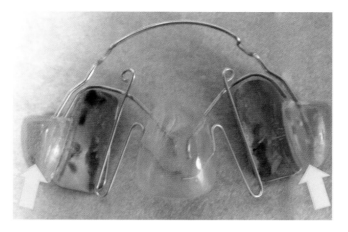

Figure 5.15 FGB appliance component: buccal shields.

is in a relaxed position, the appliance lies on the lower arch in a completely passive manner. Activation of the appliance occurs spontaneously during normal swallowing or mouth closure, events that bring the bites into contact (simultaneously) with upper and lower teeth, respecting the mandible's self-repositioning mechanism. For this reason, it can be worn both day and night, as swallowing also occurs during sleep. This produces self-regulating, rhythmic, and intermittent forces, with the same characteristics as physiological functional rhythmic movements.

The shape of the buccal shields is extremely important (Figure 5.16): they are triangular shaped with the largest mesial width that gradually decreases until it disappears distally. This shape, studied at length and refined over time, allows masseter action to be intercepted on the long side of the buccal shield and the FGB appliance to be pushed forward, creating a wedge-like action that contributes to the activation of the expansion springs (Figures 5.16 and 5.17).

5.2.1.2.2 Transmission of self-regulated muscular force to expansion
springs (Figure 5.18)

The force that activates the FGB appliance's expansion springs depends directly on the action of the muscles on the buccal shields (muscular anchorage):

- *Muscle force.* The contraction of the masseter on one side, intercepting the buccal shield, *transmits the force to the contralateral expansion spring. The thicker* the buccal shield, *the stronger the muscular pressure* transmitted to the expansion spring will be. Thus, the force of the expansion spring on the right-hand side is produced by masseteric contraction on the left against the left-hand buccal shield (opposite side to the spring) and, vice versa, the force of the expansion spring on the left-hand side is produced by masseteric contraction on the right against the right-hand buccal shield (opposite side to the spring). In other words, the force of the expansion springs may be *regulated by the thickness of the buccal shields* – the thicker they are, the greater their ability to intercept the force of masseter muscle transmitting it to the contralateral spring, on the horizontal plane. The correction is achieved gradually until the buccal cusps of the upper teeth, which were previously in crossbite, overlap the lower teeth, thus providing the appropriate physiological stimuli from peripheral receptors and proprioceptors (Figure 5.19).

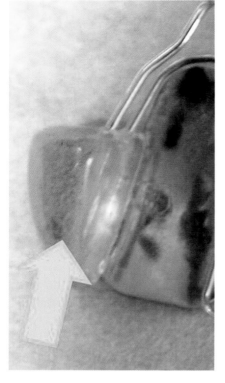

Figure 5.16 Detail of the buccal shield.

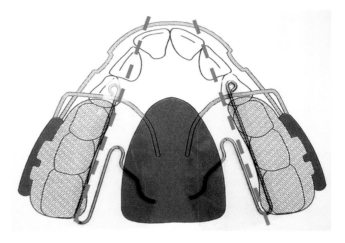

Figure 5.17 Action wedge of the buccal shield. *Source:* P. Bracco, Turin; Italy. Reproduced with permission from P. Bracco.

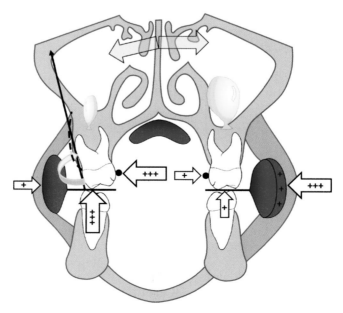

Figure 5.18 Asymmetrical action of the buccal shields for the correction of unilateral posterior crossbites.

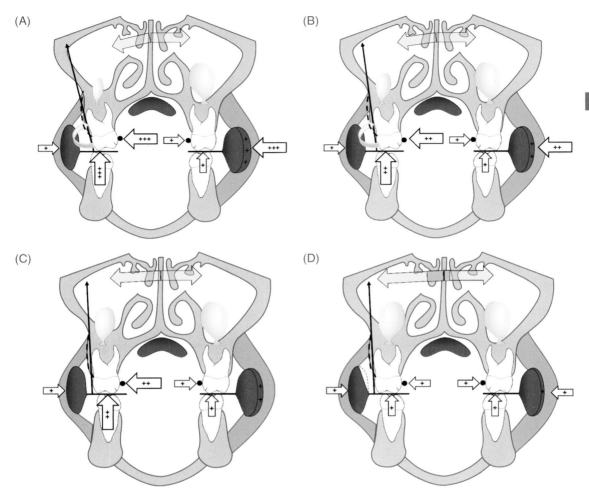

Figure 5.19 Transmission of self-regulated muscle forces to expansion springs through buccal shields for the correction of unilateral posterior crossbites. Adapting the buccal shields in an asymmetrical way, it is possible to apply asymmetrical forces and achieve true asymmetrical action during the correction of the unilateral posterior crossbite. This is an asymmetrical malocclusion requiring the possibility of application of asymmetrical forces; this is only possible with extra-dental anchorage, as with the FGB appliance that progressively works with muscular anchorage (a–d). Observe the internal and external adaptation of the buccal shields.

- *Wedge-like action.* The activation of the springs is linked also to the triangular shape of the buccal shields (thicker at the front and gradually decreasing in thickness as it moves back) which are intercepted by the muscles, *promoting the forward push of the appliance with a wedge-like action* and contributing to the activation of the expansion springs, particularly in the posterior areas. This force also works horizontally.
- *Occlusal force.* Via the bites, the occlusal force also pushes the device upward and pushes the expansion springs to equatorial tooth level, producing a bilateral expansive force which is again horizontal.

These forces are produced simultaneously and add up together to achieve an orthodontic force capable of moving teeth in a buccal direction.

The sum of these forces alone would not be capable of achieving a bodily movement as the teeth are subject to force of a sole direction, and at one single point. To avoid the application of a single force, which leads to a tilting-type movement of the teeth without stimulating bone growth and producing a significant risk of relapse, *it is necessary to apply a second force. The FGB's uniqueness,* compared with other functional appliances, *lies in its ability to produce dual force.* The *second force,* which is applied to teeth simultaneously with the expansion force, is the occlusal force. This is applied *vertically and transmitted to the teeth by the metal bite.* Thus, the horizontal force of the expansion spring (buccal shields, wedge-type action, occlusal force) and the simultaneous vertical force produced by the occlusal bite, create a dual force on teeth that leads to the *bodily repositioning of teeth.* The significance of this mechanism is not only orthodontic but also linked to the consequential *stimulation of growth and remodeling of dental-alveolar bone* in the phases of growth and development.

5.2.1.2.3 *Production of symmetric and asymmetric forces, without side effects, to achieve forces coherent with the therapeutic goals* (Figure 5.19)

As explained in Chapter 4, unilateral posterior crossbite is an asymmetric pathology and, according to the structural characteristics of the unilateral posterior crossbite, we need an appliance that is adaptable to the asymmetry of the malocclusion and to the therapeutic stage in progress. In fact, during therapy throughout the different correction stages, it is necessary to adapt the expansion spring activation process to the new occlusion. Symmetric or asymmetric activation with the FGB appliance is possible thanks to its muscular (non-dental) anchorage. We have already mentioned that masseter force on one side is transmitted via a buccal shield to the expansion spring on the other side. Thus, the expansion spring on the crossbite side receives the contralateral masseteric muscle force, which (as previously described) is characterized by a higher EMG amplitude than that of the masseter on the crossbite side, which, instead, is hypotonic and shows a smaller volume.

The FGB appliance exploits neuromuscular features effectively.

To achieve asymmetric activation (i.e. more intense on the crossbite side that needs correction, as opposed to the healthy side), we can make one side of the buccal shields thicker (i.e. the side contralateral to that of the crossbite). It is important to remember that the muscle anchorage allows the teeth to receive *an asymmetric force, avoiding side effects on other teeth.* This allows an *authentic correction of both dental and skeletal asymmetry, which is always present in unilateral crossbite, without side effects, and achieving forces coherent with the treatment objectives.* At any moment, by simply adapting the thickness of the buccal shields, it is possible to render the action and force of the appliance symmetrical, *adapting it in an appropriate manner to the therapy as it evolves.* This type of action cannot be achieved with orthodontic appliances that are anchored to teeth, where the principle reigns that each action corresponds to a similar and contrary reaction that are usually not desired side effects.

The development (via teeth) of coherent, intermittent, self-regulated, and modulated forces over time in an unrestricted system is a unique, gnathological, possibility that allows us to *cure,* in the real sense of the word, *the stomatognathic system of young patients,* producing functional equilibrium and harmonious skeletal growth. The concept that we wish to underline here is that of "curing and restoring equilibrium" via the teeth, as opposed to simply "straightening teeth." Any traumatic therapy during developmental age without attention to the function and growth may produce unpredictable and non-preventable side effects, due to the complexity of the system.

5.2.1.2.4 *Creation of decompression spaces for formation of new bone tissue and dental stability* (Figure 5.20)

Another important aspect of buccal shields is decompression, created *between the inner part of the buccal shield and the alveolar bone.* The buccal shield must always be distinctly

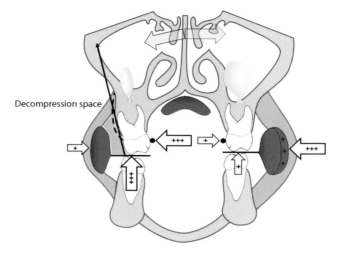

Figure 5.20   Decompression space, represented in gray.

detached from the alveolar bone, and in this way, creating a decompression space where the muscle is no longer in contact with the bone but is sustained by the shield, it promotes the formation and apposition of new bone, which is important for future stability.

5.2.1.2.5 Anchorage of the arches and optionals

Furthermore, buccal shields provide anchorage for the arches, which may be fixed in such a way as to produce contact with the incisors of the upper arch (class II buccal arch) or those of the lower arch (class III buccal arch). Apart from the buccal arches, which are an integral part of the appliance, optional buccal shields can be anchored, such as upper (for class III malocclusions) or lower (for class II) lip-bumper buccal arches. These create a decompression space in front of the alveolar bone of the incisors, allowing its continued growth. We mention these optionals for functionalizing devices because they can, if necessary, be used alongside and simultaneously with the crossbite correction.

5.2.1.3 *Expansion springs* (Figure 5.21)

Actions and effects:

1. Forces transmitted by the expansion springs.
2. Diametric increase of the intermolar distance.
3. Remodeling and symmetric resetting of the basal development.

Expansion springs are a vital component of the FGB appliance, especially when correcting unilateral posterior crossbite. In the past, they were considered an optional element, but research has proven that they provide a fundamental contribution to the overall efficiency of the appliance. The condition most suited to the use of expansion springs is posterior crossbite, particularly when unilateral (i.e. in the pathology that benefits most from intermittent tensile expansion force). However, in all other cases also, this easily adopted option *optimizes the appliance's performance by means of intermittent, tensile forces*.

These springs are anchored to the palatal button and must be positioned, in passive conditions with the mandible at rest, 2 mm below the tooth equator.

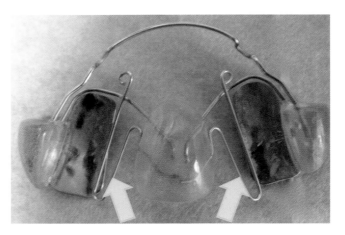

Figure 5.21 FGB appliance component: expansion springs.

5.2.1.3.1 Forces transmitted by the expansion springs

During activity (deglutition), the expansion spring is pushed to the level of the tooth equator, transmitting an expansive elastic, tensile force in a horizontal direction. Thanks to its shape, it transmits an elastic force to teeth, via punctiform contacts. As explained previously, the expansion springs are activated by masseteric pressure and not by a direct activation of the spring which, during therapy, only needs to be repositioned 2 mm under the teeth equator. We report here again the activation of the expansion spring:

- *Muscle force*. The contraction of the masseter on one side, intercepting the buccal shield, *transmits the force to the contralateral expansion spring. The thicker* the buccal shield, *the stronger the muscular pressure* transmitted to the expansion spring will be. Thus, the force of the expansion spring on the right-hand side is produced by masseteric contraction on the left against the left-hand buccal shield (opposite side to the spring) and, vice versa, the force of the expansion spring on the left-hand side is produced by masseteric contraction on the right against the right-hand buccal shield (opposite side to the spring). In other words, the force of the expansion springs may be *regulated by the thickness of the buccal shields* – the thicker they are, the greater their ability to intercept the force of masseter muscle transmitting it to the contralateral spring, on the horizontal plane. This force is intermittent, tensile, and self-regulating.
- *Wedge-like action*. The activation of the springs is linked also to the triangular shape of the buccal shields (thicker at the front and gradually decreasing in thickness as it moves back) which are intercepted by the muscles, *promoting the forward push of the appliance with a wedge-like action* and contributing to the activation of the expansion springs, particularly in the posterior areas. This force also works horizontally and intermittent, tensile, and self-regulating.
- *Occlusal force*. Via the bites, the occlusal force also pushes the device upward and pushes the expansion springs to equatorial tooth level, producing a bilateral expansive force, which is again horizontal, intermittent, tensile, and self-regulating.

These forces are produced simultaneously and add up together to achieve an orthodontic, intermittent, tensile force capable of moving teeth in a buccal direction.

Thus, the force is physiological because it acts respecting the sutures and structures biology and is self-regulating.

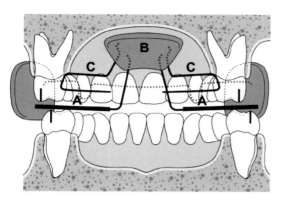 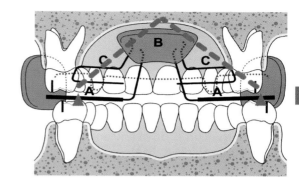

Figure 5.22   Intermittent forces; activation of the appliance during swallowing. A: resilient stainless steel bite planes; B: palatal button; C: expansion springs. *Source:* Piancino *et al.* (2006).

To sum up, the expansion springs are activated by:

1. the buccal shields, which intercept the masseter muscle and transmit the force to the contralateral expansion spring;
2. the wedge-type action of the buccal shields;
3. the occlusal force, which pushes the appliance upward and takes the expansion springs to the same level as the tooth equator, activating it with intermittent and expansive elastic force (Figure 5.22).

As explained earlier, all these forces work horizontally, and if the expansion spring were the only source of force applied to the teeth (as usually occurs with removable orthodontic appliances) there would simply be a tilting movement with hardly any stimulation of bone growth. With the FGB appliance, on the other hand, *a second force is applied vertically to teeth, via the bite, allowing bodily movement of teeth* (Figure 5.23). The resilient stainless steel bite planes, which we previously described, simultaneously level the occlusal plane, align the dental arches, and transmit force to the teeth and roots.

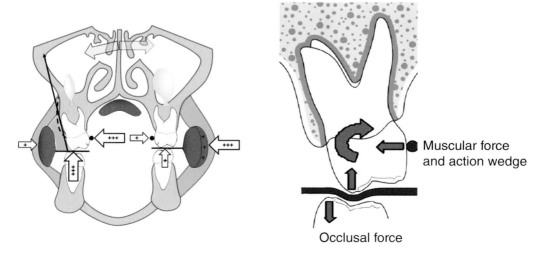

Muscular force and action wedge

Occlusal force

Figure 5.23   The simultaneous actions of the FGB appliance realize bodily movement of the teeth. The decompression space is represented in grey.

The bodily movement allows a *repositioning of the tooth and its root within the alveolar bone, stimulating growth and remodeling* of the support bone. On the contrary, the tilting movement caused by the application of a single force creates the potential for a relapse into dental malposition and does not stimulate bone growth (which is, however, one of the most important goals of interceptive orthodontic treatment). Here, we should also remember the role of decompression spaces, which promote the apposition of alveolar bone and react synergistically.

As well as stimulating and remodeling the local alveolar bone, the *action of the expansion springs* (important for restoring harmony to bone growth) *is carried out in the palate via dental roots*. Regarding physiological growth, we have already seen the importance of the transmittance of forces via the roots of first molars during mastication. Similarly, thanks to its wedge-type action, its intermittent occlusal force that pushes the expansion springs to the equator level of teeth, and the force transmitted by buccal shields, the functionalizing appliance contributes to the *tensile forces on the palatal suture, which have been proven to be the physiological forces for stimulation of bone apposition respecting the viscoelastic properties of the sutures*. We will examine this topic in depth later, but here we would like to underline that the orthodontic action of the functionalizing appliance is entirely absent of any dental or bone traumatism and that it is inserted into the stomatognathic system in line with its physiological characteristics; that is, along the same principles as the function – avoiding traumatism but promoting intermittent and tensile forces calibrated individually by muscles, decompression spaces, cuspid protection, and self-repositioning of the mandible. Furthermore, during orthodontic movement of teeth, which is an acute stage (in the sense that the occlusal situation can alter in various areas simultaneously and in a short time period) and at risk of traumatic contacts, with FGB occlusion is protected and the mandible is constantly disengaged and self-repositioned in a centered position. This means that, even during orthodontic movement, the system is protected from traumatic contacts, balanced from a muscular point of view and never forced.

5.2.1.3.2 *Diametric increase of the intermolar distance* (Figure 5.24)

The *intercanine and intermolar diametric increase of the upper arch is the consequence* not only of the dental movement, but also *of alveolar and palatal growth*, thanks to the action mechanisms already explained.

One important action of the FGB appliance that, via the teeth, harmony is restored to bone growth and, as explained, masticatory function is rebalanced. Therefore, the goal of orthodontic treatment with an FGB appliance, especially during childhood, is not simple dental repositioning but *a true restoral of physiological function to the stomatognathic system, masticatory function, and growth*. The achievement of this goal with the FGB appliance was refined over years of research (Bracco *et al.*, 1979; Piancino *et al.*, 2006). It is useful to remember that to obtain these results it is necessary to understand the action mechanisms of the appliance in order to *plan* (diagnosis and choice of most suitable FGB), *realize* (laboratory technique), and *adjust and activate* (clinically) in the *most appropriate manner*.

Moreover, to achieve and maintain the correct arch diameters (supported by the growth of dentoalveolar bone and palate) it is important to give the right level of stimulation to growth at the right time. *Initial correction* requires maximum collaboration, and must and can be achieved *in the briefest time possible*. However, *it would be a mistake* to consider the correction of a serious growth altered condition such as unilateral posterior crossbite in a short period and *without follow-up maintenance*.

Initial dental correction, which we may consider to be an active counter-step, lasts on average 4–8 months (depending on age, gravity of the malocclusion, and the patient's structural features). Following this, the device should be worn at home and during the night (or during the night only), allowing the child to continue the restoration of correct masticatory function and

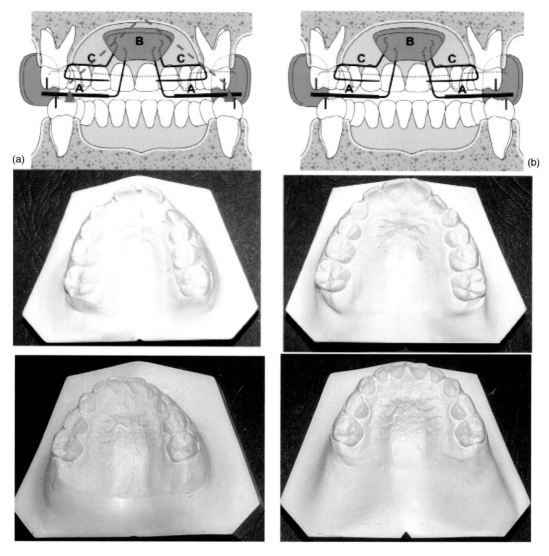

Figure 5.24 Narrow and asymmetrical palatal vault before therapy (a); observe the expansion of the palatal vault, but especially the recovery of the asymmetry (b) after therapy with FGB appliance in mixed (*top*) and deciduous dentition (*bottom*). A: resilient stainless steel bite planes; B: palatal button; C: expansion springs.

balanced growth over time. This possibility, which eases life for the patient, is important because it allows the arch and occlusion improvement over time according to the ideal form of the appliance. Any anomalous eruption of a new tooth can be repaired with a simple adjustment of the expansion spring before the tooth even enters into an occlusal condition, thus avoiding wrong contacts. In fact, as the appliance does not have dental anchorage, its use can be continued even during the transition period, when it is possible to provide *early correction of any anomalous eruptions*.

5.2.1.3.3 *Remodeling and symmetric resetting of the basal development*

The symmetric resetting and harmonious rebalancing of palatal bone growth are just some of the important results of an FGB appliance, both generally and specifically for the correction of unilateral posterior crossbite. In fact, as already mentioned, this appliance (by means of teeth and roots) creates tensile forces *on the palatal suture, in full respect of the vascularization and viscoelastic properties of the suture*, which are important aspects regarding the stimulation of the palatal bone growth.

Furthermore, the appliance allows both symmetric and asymmetric activation, an important factor in the correction of unilateral posterior crossbite. Simple expansion without targeted actions on teeth and bone is not enough, as correction of the asymmetries of the malocclusion is the real aim of the early therapy. We know that this is a malocclusion characterized by asymmetry that manifests as a dental malocclusion, but it is the consequence of asymmetric function and growth from the earliest stages of development. The asymmetric features linked to unilateral posterior crossbite are easily identified in patients, both within the stomatognathic system and in posture. A targeted therapy is necessary to correct the asymmetry. When the expansion is symmetric in an asymmetric structure, the asymmetry will not be corrected, it will be stabilized over time.

The correction of crossbite conditions can be achieved over a short period of time, but in the light of everything described above, it would be a mistake to abandon patients with this type of malocclusion after treatment at a mere dental level without considering all the other aspects of "crossbite syndrome," which require longer times for physiological and stable treatment. With an FGB appliance, this can be easily achieved by wearing it at home and at night, or solely at night but with constancy, and leaving the child free to leave it off for the rest of the day. Here, we would like to underline the importance, during childhood, of active physiological maintenance that neither forces nor restricts the system in any way, in order to achieve harmonious structural growth. The FGB appliance "works for us," enabling us to "cure" the stomatognathic system of young patients, in the knowledge that the future equilibrium of the stomatognathic system is important for the future quality of life.

The correction of this entirely asymmetric malocclusion with dental anchorage mechanisms that exert pressure on the system and develop predetermined symmetric forces is certainly not ideal because it does not correct asymmetry and, above all, because it requires true mandibular compensation. The question thus may arise here: is it really necessary to worry about such a complex system overall? Could we not just concentrate on "straightening" teeth, in the hope that everything else will "set itself right"? With the neuromuscular knowledge currently at our disposal, we know well that "almost nothing will fix itself" – on the contrary, the risk of future imbalances in patients inclined toward facial pain will instead increase; and as things stand today, we have no possibility of previously identifying these patients. The goal of precocious orthodontic treatment cannot be simply "adjustment" without any biological or physiological grounding, but must instead be aimed at restoration of function and growth, based on scientific evidence and knowledge to lower the risk of future imbalance.

5.2.1.4 *Palatal button* (Figure 5.25)

Actions and effects:

1. Re-education of the tongue.
2. Stabilization.
3. Anchorage of the expansion springs and optionals.

The palatal button of the FGB appliance has an important action on the tongue function.

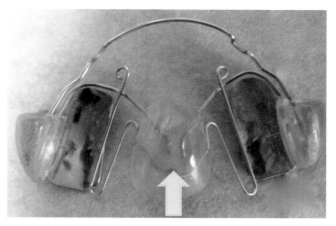

Figure 5.25 FGB appliance component: palatal button.

5.2.1.4.1 *Re-education of the tongue* (Figure 5.26)

The re-education of the tongue occurs thanks to the fact that the *palatal button*, also referred to as the "artificial bolus" by P. Bracco, acts in the same way as *a real food bolus*, drawing the tongue to it and *refunctionalizing the mechanism of deglutition*, as outlined in Garliner's sequence of deglutition (Garliner, 1976; Schindler *et al.*, 2011). The normalizing of the peristaltic action of deglutition causes the patient to push (automatically and effortlessly) the tongue against the palate as opposed to the teeth. This is an irreplaceable logopedic action with effects on deglutition, phonation, and so on. The *neuromuscular rebalancing* of agonist and antagonist muscles, such as the tongue and lips, is fundamental for *stable orthodontic correction*. We know that the position of teeth is a result of muscular equilibrium. The simple volume of the tongue and its placement can influence the growth and position of skeletal structures. *The force vectors of the tongue are repetitive and cyclical* – owing to this fact, when not controlled, they can contribute to the emergence of the worst malocclusions, particularly on the vertical plane.

(a)   (b)

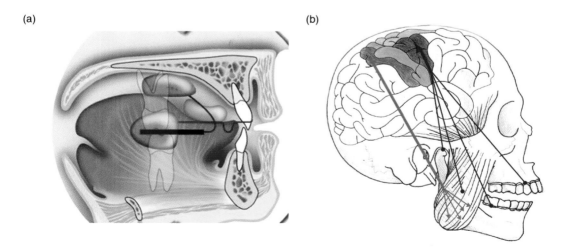

Figure 5.26 The palatal button acts as an artificial bolus (a). Restoration of the tongue function and swallowing automatism (b).

5.2.1.4.2 Stabilization

The stabilization action of the palatal button takes place because, as the tongue is drawn to it, it pushes the device against the palate, stabilizing it and preparing it for the next action of occlusal force that will occur via the metal bites. It is clear that, for this action to take place, the appliance must be correctly set up, with a space of approximately 2 mm between the palate and the palatal button.

5.2.1.4.3 Anchorage of the expansion springs and optionals

Furthermore, the palatal button represents a point of anchorage of the wires and springs.

5.2.2 Histomorphological issues of the palatal suture as a biological basis for the action of the Function Generating Bite appliance

The rehabilitation of a complex function such as mastication and of an equally complex development such as cranial growth calls for specific and appropriate methods of treatment. *Any major invasive intervention on cranial structures during childhood will have unpredictable and non-preventable results* (Stevens *et al.*, 2011; Muchitsch *et al.*, 2012; Bazargani *et al.*, 2013). Fortunately, such interventions are no longer necessary (even though they continue to be commonly adopted), as they are unsupported by any physiological or biological needs. We have described how the expansive action of the FGB appliance is characterized by intermittent and self-regulated forces, and how these forces are transmitted via teeth to skeletal structures. Regarding this issue, we would like to cite some histological and molecular research studies that explain the physiological reasons behind the action mechanisms of the FGB appliance.

One author who has made an important contribution to this field (from both histological and clinical points of view) is B. Thilander, who demonstrated *the importance of mastication and bolus consistency, which means transmission of muscular forces via the teeth, for the development and active apposition of bone in the palatal suture during growth* (Figure 5.27). In experimental studies on rats fed with soft food compared with those fed with normal food, the first group clearly displayed a narrower, less active, and almost calcified palatal suture (Kiliaridis *et al.*, 1985; Engström *et al.*, 1986) (Figure 5.28b)

On the basis of studies using rabbits and human autopsy remains, it emerged that the palatal suture in both cases was characterized by high vascularization and that the growth took place without the participation of cartilaginous tissue but via ossification. Moreover, the tensile forces (typical of an FGB appliance) stimulate the *formation of collagenous bands* that foster osteogenesis and may be viewed as the precursor of autogenous bone grafting (Persson *et al.*, 1978).

More recently, it was confirmed that sutures produce new bone at the sutural edges of the bone fronts in response to external stimuli. To function as bone growth sites, sutures need to remain patent, while allowing rapid bone formation at the edges of the bone fronts (Hinton, 1988; Opperman, 2000; Katsaros, 2001).

These results are supported by those conclusions regarding the timing of calcification (Rice, 2008):

> *Most facial sutures remain patent until late adulthood. For example, the frontomaxillary, nasomaxillary and zygomaticomaxillary sutures do not start to fuse until the 7th or 8th decade of life. This is presumably due to mechanical strain*

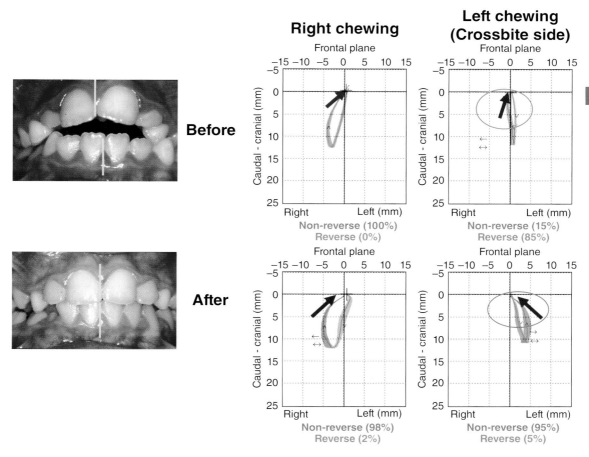

Figure 5.30 Recovery of the chewing pattern before/after therapy with FGB appliance of a patient with anterior open bite and left unilateral posterior crossbite.

normalization of the system. This is the first vital result that is achieved with biological and physiological therapy. However, the recovery of reverse closure is just the first step, and to allow the pattern to improve it is necessary to continue the work of the FGB appliance, gradually, to give the neuromuscular system the time to reprogram itself in a stable way.

The high significance of results achieved by comparing the number of reverse cycles before and after treatment with an FGB appliance shows that the phenomenon is clear and repeatable. The *control of masticatory function*, which is easily achieved with the use of electrognathography, is important as it demonstrates whether the therapeutic goal of functional recovery has been achieved. Furthermore, it allows an early diagnosis of which patients suffer greater difficulty in normalizing function and are therefore more at risk of relapse. This allows us, first of all, to identify such patients and follow them more carefully, modifying and adapting the functionalizing treatment as necessary. As electrognathography is a non-invasive examination, it can easily be repeated more times in order to check the functional change.

5.2.5 Cranial–maxillofacial basal actions and effects of the Function Generating Bite appliance

This section will examine the action of the appliance on dynamic posture of the mandible and *its effects on cranial growth as a whole*. This topic is complex but is fundamental in order to understand the vectorial characteristics and action mechanisms of functionalizing appliances.

First of all, we would like to underline the *importance of cephalometry as a diagnostic tool*. We have already explained that teeth are an integral part of a complex system, and without the aid of cephalometry it is not possible to make a precise diagnosis or select the most suitable therapy. However, traditional cephalometry (i.e., morphological, structural, and static analysis of the cranium) has *evolved into dynamic-functional analysis*, identifying the *functional vectors* that act on and *influence the growth of cranial structure* (Figure 5.31).

In fact, it is from vectorial analysis that we understand *the negative dynamics that are established when cranial morphology varies from the mean*. Vectors and negative dynamics are related to gnathological functional changes; by understanding these, we are able to choose and adopt therapies targeted at neutralization of those vectors responsible for abnormal muscle and joint loads. For this reason we have superimposed the "motor" of function (i.e., the muscles) on cephalometric tracing. Looking at their relation to bone structure it is easy to understand the force vectors generated by the masseter, one of the most important masticatory muscles. It clearly shows how different force vectors of muscles can be, according to cranial typology (Figure 5.31).

Traditional orthodontics previously awarded great importance to skeletal classification on the sagittal plane, with diagnosis and therapies aimed at treating classes I/II/III conditions. Currently, we know that *pathologies which produce negative dynamic vectors*, thus harming skeletal growth and, particularly, TMJ development, are *linked to changes on the vertical dimension and frontal plane*.

The alterations *on the vertical plane* create vectors that condition the dynamic posture of the mandible, the occlusal plane, and the TMJ, influencing morphological development. The alterations *on the frontal plane concern asymmetrical growth and occlusion, and create asymmetric* functional dynamic vectors that cause the skeletal asymmetry to become even worse and lead to unharmonious growth patterns between the two sides. *In both cases, at the end of growth, the consequences of pathological vectors are irreversible*. To improve the functioning of the system, treatment has to be started during childhood/development, based on an accurate diagnosis, aimed to improve cranial vectors.

From this point of view, functionalizing appliances are of great help because, if chosen and designed correctly, they improve the vertical structure and mandible dynamics at the same time as correcting the asymmetric conditions described earlier. Regarding the vertical dimension, it is important to remember that it is directly linked to the dynamic posture of the mandible and to the force vectors that act on TMJ movement during function and growth.

In hyperdivergent cases (Figure 5.32), the *growth direction of the mandible is clockwise* and the muscle forces are characterized by vectors that tend to constantly shift (during any type of function) the condyle and the meniscus forward. These negative forces are an intrinsic feature of the cranial structure in hyperdivergent cases and lead to a constant backward rotation of the mandible and to a clockwise-sense growth with varying possibilities of anteriorization of the condylar–meniscal complex. It is clearly important to choose a therapeutic solution that does not strengthen these negative vectors but, if possible, neutralizes or counteracts them.

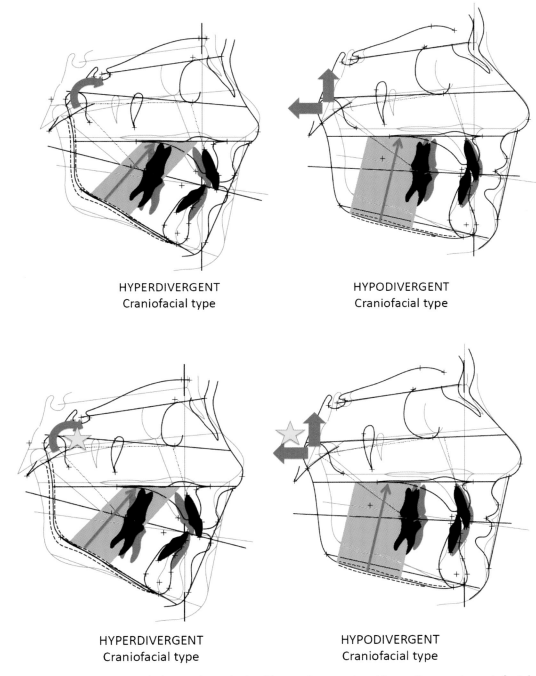

HYPERDIVERGENT
Craniofacial type

HYPODIVERGENT
Craniofacial type

HYPERDIVERGENT
Craniofacial type

HYPODIVERGENT
Craniofacial type

Figure 5.31   Dynamic cephalometric analysis of hyperdivergent and hypodivergent craniofacial morphology with muscular and articular vector of forces represented.

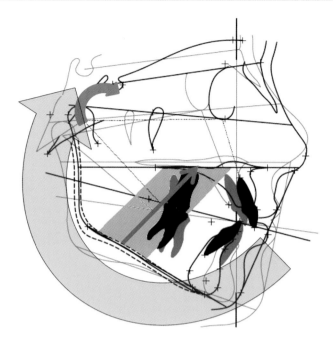

Figure 5.32 Dynamic cephalometric analysis in the sagittal plane of a hyperdivergent craniofacial morphology with mandibular clockwise vector of forces represented in red.

The posterior bites of the FGB appliance serve to pull the mandible downward, neutralizing negative vectors on the condylar–meniscal complex and promoting the repositioning and growth in an anti-clockwise direction of the mandible (Figure 5.33). The posterior metal bites allow the mandible to self-reposition in the three spatial planes, but, above all, thanks to the masseteric force, they inhibit the dentoalveolar bone of the posterior sectors, favoring the growth of the mandible with forward mandibular rotation and dynamic posture in an anti-clockwise direction. In this way, the bites neutralize the pathological vectors that, in the absence of any corrective appliance, perform in a clockwise sense. Thus, simultaneously with its orthodontic dental repositioning action, the FGB appliance also has actions and effects in the three spatial planes that work against the negative dynamic vectors, improving the function and structural growth of young patients still in the period of development.

We have described hyperdivergent cranial structure because it is often linked to crossbite conditions and is the most difficult to deal with in orthodontics, involving more potential collateral damage.

Obviously, there are also cases of opposite cranial structure (hypodivergent), which require an appliance with the opposite features. The direction of mandibular growth in these cases is anti-clockwise, the opposite of those that are hyperdivergent, and the vector forces generally tend to shift the condyle backward and upward. These intrinsic negative forces of hypodivergent cranial structures are combated with functionalizing devices with anterior bites that generally reposition and promote mandible growth in a clockwise sense, neutralizing the negative anti-clockwise vectors of hypodivergent cranial structures (Figure 5.34).

It is clear that the earlier the FGB appliance is adopted, the greater the chances of success will be in modifying and rebalancing cranial growth and TMJ development and remodeling.

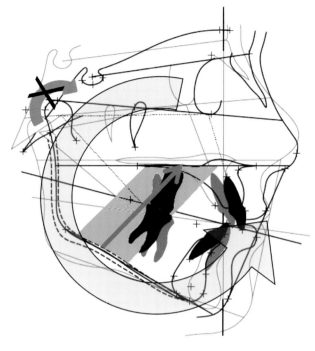

Figure 5.33 Representation of counter-clockwise vector of forces (green) generated by the posterior stainless steel resilient bite planes of FGB in a hyperdivergent subject, counteracting the vectors on the TMJ.

(a)   (b)

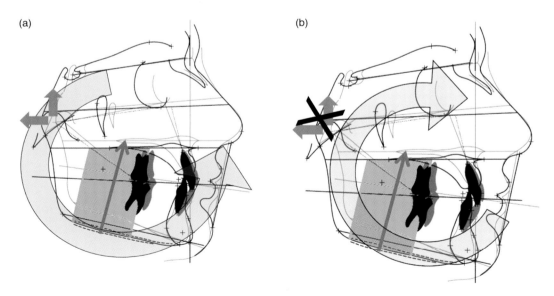

Figure 5.34 Dynamic cephalometric analysis of hypodivergent subject with counter-clockwise vector of forces (red) (a); representation of clockwise vector of forces (green) generated by FGB anterior and posterior bite planes (b), lowering the TMJ overload.

For this reason, the influence of the functionalizing device on joint function has been carefully studied. We published an article on the subject, in collaboration with R. Slavicek, showing that there is significant recovery of condylar tracings registered in axiographic tracking records before and after functionalizing treatment. The patients analyzed all suffered from cranial–mandibular disorders and were subdivided into a group of young/developing patients and a group at the end of the growth period (Piancino et al., 2008). Functional improvement was highlighted in both groups, but the childhood/developing group not only demonstrated *a stronger recovery of condylar shifts but also recovered asymmetric tracks, in contrast with the group at the end of the growth period, who showed no significant result from this point of view* (Figure 5.35).

This is due to the fact that asymmetric tracks are the result of anatomically asymmetric structures, which can only be repaired at prepubescent age with the use of functionalizing devices. At the end of the growth, it may still be possible to improve functional movements, but the anatomical structure itself is impossible to modify.

We know that the TMJ is totally undeveloped at birth, and that it will undergo vital changes during development; even more importantly, it is characterized by *an adaptive type of growth* (Ingervall et al., 1976; Thilander et al., 1976). This feature is of great importance. On one hand, the plasticity and adaptability of the TMJ allows the "rebalancing" of growth and joint structures (impossible during adulthood) (Piancino et al., 2008); on the other hand, the use of the wrong device can worsen the imbalance in function and growth. This is why disengagement of the mandible, muscle anchorage, intermittent forces, and self-regulation of functionalizing appliances prevent undesirable side effects and offer the possibility of orthognathodontic therapy aimed at truly recovering static and dynamic equilibrium of the entire stomatognathic system.

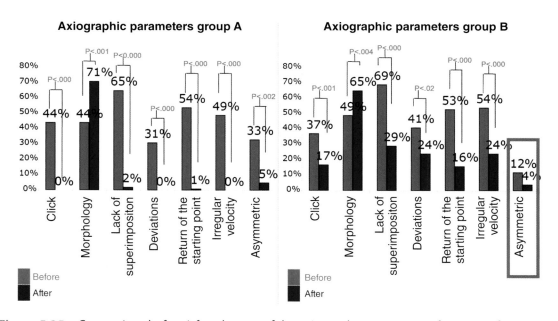

Figure 5.35 Comparison before/after therapy of the axiography parameters of a group of young/developing patients (group A) with a group at the end of the growth period (group B). The only non-significant parameter is the asymmetry of tracing in the group at the end of the growth period (see text for explanation).

Thus, the functionalizing device is able to combat negative vectors linked to the developing cranial structure and to correct asymmetry at the same time.

Regarding the interception of class II and III pathologies on the sagittal plane, the functionalizing appliances (as previously mentioned) feature class II/III buccal arches, upper/lower buccal shields, and other optionals. These optionals act to improve harmonious growth of the maxillaries via the creation of compression and decompression areas. The issue of functionalizing appliances with anterior bites and the use of optional features will be examined in later updates – we believe it necessary to briefly mention the topic in this book to clarify to the reader that FGB appliances have been fine-tuned over the years on the basis of clinical experience, and that they may be specifically customized for all types of cranial structures and dental malocclusions in light of the best orthognathodontic therapies. In the same way, it would be useful to look further at the characteristics of posture and scapular belts, topics that border on other disciplines and feature in multidisciplinary studies. We are well aware of the connections and importance of these issues, which will be the topic of a future study with particular focus on the actions and effects of FGB appliances.

5.3 Therapy timing and duration and caries-free management

FGB appliances are activated during phonation and deglutition. They are recommended for *early treatment of malocclusions characterized by functional alteration of the stomatognathic system*, such as unilateral posterior crossbite, which unequivocally modifies masticatory function, or dental open bite, which alters the functional behavior of the tongue and deglutition. Modification of function is the cause/effect of these types of malocclusion and is responsible for the ingravescence (the continual worsening) of functional imbalance. These are malocclusions that need correction "as early as possible" during the phase of growth in order to achieve re-equilibrium of function during childhood. Of course, the *first stage of treatment* must adapt to *the psychophysical needs of the child*, as the "age of development" offers a wider range of solutions; but, at the same time, *the more time that passes, the more the system adjusts gradually yet irreversibly to the malocclusion.*

Regarding the correct time to start treatment, for crossbite the use of an FGB appliance is generally recommended as soon as possible. If the family is willing, a crossbite condition can be fixed, even during deciduous dentition. At this age, the correction is carried out extremely quickly. The first stage of mixed dentition, following the eruption of permanent first molars and incisors, is a period still suitable for therapeutic intervention with FGB appliances for functional and structural purposes. As the growth stage progresses, structural repair becomes increasingly difficult. However, each case needs to be evaluated individually, adjusting therapy times as appropriate.

Regarding the use of FGB appliances over time, it is important to remember that, from the initial phase until the final correction of dental malocclusion, the appliance must be worn "as much as possible." It is recommended that the dental correction (or rather the "hypercorrection") be achieved as quickly as possible. As soon as the dental condition is satisfactory (generally following 4–8 months of treatment), use of the FGB appliance can be limited to home and nighttime. It would be a mistake to suspend the therapy at this point simply because dental correction has been achieved, as dental irregularity is only one small part of a much wider pathology. The system must be allowed sufficient time to repair static and dynamic imbalances, which require attention over time in full respect of normal physiological conditions. Thus, during the second stage, the device will be worn at home and at night (or solely at night, depending on the seriousness of the case). The FGB appliance can be used over time, where necessary, to promote balanced growth without collateral effects, in full respect of physiological and biological wellbeing, *and with stable results*. In fact, FGB appliances, differently from appliances with dental anchorage, can be used over time, lightly continuing the expansion activity during growth, to the great advantage of the patient.

From this point of view, it is important to underline the fact that the appliance (without any form of dental anchorage) can support the *eruption of new teeth without the need for modification* and that *ectopic eruptions*, should they occur, can be *corrected* with just a simple adjustment of the expansion springs, *even before the tooth enters an occlusal position and in function*.

The overall treatment times vary, obviously, according to the case at hand, the cranial structure, and the seriousness of the malocclusion.

Finally, it is important to underline that by avoiding dental anchorage in favor of punctiform-type contacts, *the FGB appliance may be classified as entirely noncariogenic*. This is an important factor considering that the appliance is used in the childhood period of growth, when dental hygiene is often less than perfect and toothbrushing techniques are still generally in need of improvement.

It is high on our list of priorities to develop therapies that fulfill the fundamental principle of medicine – *primum non nocere* – and we can safely say that the FGB appliance obeys this principle from protective, orthodontic, and gnathological points of view.

5.4 Compliance

Last but not least, another important point to outline, understand, and evaluate in the use of this device is the level of collaboration from the patient. We know that there is no successful orthodontic treatment without the willing collaboration of the patient. The concept, which leads a large number of orthodontists and manufacturing companies to select a "no compliance" appliance, is based on mechanical factors as opposed to physiological factors and their relevant consequences. The stomatognathic system is one of the most refined and complex structures in the human body, which develops over a period spanning from 0 to 20 years. These two characteristics (complexity and duration of development) require a therapy in full physiological respect of the stomatognathic system, on which the patient's quality of life depends.

When the doctor is fully aware of how important the choice of therapy is for the patient, he/she will be able to explain the reasons behind this choice and to motivate the patients, gaining their full cooperation and trust in the treatment process.

One last consideration from an organizational point of view: the work undertaken in the dental chair certainly requires competence in medicine and biology, but it calls for relatively limited time in a practical sense as the technical activation of the FGB appliance is relatively simple, thus easing the work of the dental/orthodontic practice. FGB appliances really work for us.

The orthognathodontic therapy must then be planned according to the type of malocclusion at hand, the growth trend, and the patient's own unique characteristics in full respect of the system's physiology and biology, avoiding trauma and harmful side effects. This is how the FGB concept works, preventing relapse and achieving a balanced stomatognathic system that will allow our young patients to face the world and its problems confidently and in a determined manner. But this is also our satisfaction, in the knowledge that we have "cured" our patients, giving them not only improved aesthetic features, but especially a healthy function and harmonious growth balanced living.

References

Abed GS, Buschang PH, Taylor R, Hinton RJ. (2007) Maturational and functional related differences in rat craniofacial growth. *Arch Oral Biol* 52(11), 1018–1025.

Bazargani F, Feldmann I, Bondemark L (2013) Three-dimensional analysis of effects of rapid maxillary expansion on facial sutures and bones. A systematic review. *Angle Orthod* 83(6), 1074–1082.

Bracco P, Piancino MG. (2009) La riabilitazione occlusale con l'ortognatodonzia funzionale. In: *Elementi di gnatologia. Dalla diagnosi alla riabilitazione*, vol. 2 (eds E Tanteri, A Bracco, R Prandi). RC Libri Srl, Milan, pp. 105–514.

Bracco P, Solinas GF. (1979a) Orthognathic correction of uni- and bilateral crossbite with a functional appliance. *Mondo Ortod* 4(2), 8–24.

Bracco P, Solinas GF. (1979b) Use and control of the "function bite plate" in the early treatment of crossbite. *Mondo Ortod* 4(4), 7–17.

Castroflorio T, Talpone F, Deregibus A, *et al.* (2004) Effects of a functional appliance on masticatory muscles of young adults suffering from muscle-related temporomandibular disorders. *J Oral Rehabil* 31(6), 524–529.

Gorbonos M, Kubodera T, Rabie B, Preston B (eds). (2013) *Handbook for modern functional treatment approaches and techniques*. Ripano Editorial Medica, Madrid.

Deshayes M-J. (2006) *L'art de traiter avant 6 ans*. Éditions CRANEXPLO.

Duterloo HS, Enlow DH. (1970) A comparative study of cranial growth in *Homo* and *Macaca*. *Am J Anat* 127(4), 357–367.

Enlow DH, Bang S. (1965) Growth and remodeling of the human maxilla. *Am J Orthod* 51, 446–464.

Enlow DH (eds). (1990) *Facial growth*, 3rd edn. SPCK, University of Michigan.

Engström C, Kiliaridis S, Thilander B. (1986) The relationship between masticatory function and craniofacial morphology. II. A histological study in the growing rat fed a soft diet. *Eur J Orthod* 8(4), 271–279.

Fuentes MA, Opperman LA, Buschang P, *et al.* (2003) Lateral functional shift of the mandible: part I. Effects on condylar cartilage thickness and proliferation. *Am J Orthod Dentofacial Orthop* 123(2), 153–159.

Garliner D (ed.). (1976) *Myofunctional therapy*. WB Saunders, Philadelphia, PA.

Herring S. (2008) Mechanical influences on suture development and patency. In: *Craniofacial sutures. Development, disease and treatment* (ed. DP Rice). Karger, Basel, pp. 41–56.

Hinton RJ. (1988) Response of the intermaxillary suture cartilage to alterations in masticatory function. *Anat Rec* 220(4), 376–387.

Hinton RJ. (2014) Genes that regulate morphogenesis and growth of the temporomandibular joint: a review. *Dev Dyn* 243(7), 864–874.

Hinton RJ, Carlson DS. (1986) Response of the mandibular joint to loss of incisal function in the rat. *Acta Anat* 125(3), 145–151.

Ingervall B, Carlsson GE, Thilander B. (1976) Postnatal development of the human temporomandibular joint. II. A microradiographic study. *Acta Odontol Scand* 34(3), 133–139.

Jing J, Hinton RJ, Mishina Y, *et al.* (2014a) Critical role of Bmpr1a in mandibular condyle growth. *Connect Tissue Res* 55(Suppl 1), 73–78.

Jing J, Hinton RJ, Jing Y, *et al.* (2014b) Osterix couples chondrogenesis and osteogenesis in post-natal condylar growth. *J Dent Res* 93(10), 1014–1021.

Katsaros C. (2001) Masticatory muscle function and transverse dentofacial growth. *Swed Dent J Suppl* 151, 1–47.

Kiliaridis S, Engstrom C, Thilander B. (1985) The relationship between masticatory function and craniofacial morphology. I. A cephalometric longitudinal analysis in the growing rat fed a soft diet. *Eur J Orthod* 7(4), 273–283.

McNamara JA, Carlson DS. (1979) Quantitative analysis of temporomandibular joint adaptations to protrusive function. *Am J Orthod* 76(6), 593–611.

Moss ML, Salentijn L. (1969a) The primary role of functional matrices in facial growth. *Am J Orthod* 55(6), 566–577.

Moss ML, Salentijn L. (1969b) The capsular matrix. *Am J Orthod* 56(5), 474–490.

Muchitsch AP, Winsauer U, Wendl B, *et al.* (2012) Remodelling of the palatal dome following rapid maxillary expansion (RME): laser scan-quantifications during a low growth period. *Orthod Craniofac Res* 15(1), 30–38.

Neff P. (1999) *TMJ occlusion and function.* http://peterneffdds.com/blog, http://www.amazon.com/TMJ-occlusion-function-Peter-Neff/dp/B0006RE5SK (accessed October 2, 2015).

Opperman LA. (2000) Cranial sutures as intramembranous bone growth sites. *Dev Dyn* 219(4), 472–485.

Persson M, Magnusson BC, Thilander B. (1978) Sutural closure in rabbit and man: a morphological and histochemical study. *J Anat* 125, 313–321.

Petren S, Bjerklin K, Bondemark L. (2011) Stability of unilateral posterior crossbite correction in the mixed dentition: a randomized clinical trial with a 3-year follow-up. *Am J Orthod Dentofacial Orthop* 139(1), e73–e81.

Piancino MG, Talpone F, Dalmasso P, *et al.* (2006) Reverse-sequencing chewing patterns before and after treatment of children with a unilateral posterior crossbite. *Eur J Orthod* 28(5), 480–484.

Piancino MG, Roberi L, Frongia G, *et al.* (2008) Computerized axiography in TMD patients before and after therapy with "function generating bites". *J Oral Rehabil* 35(2), 88–94.

Purves D, Augustine GJ, Fitzpatrick, *et al.* (2000) *Neuroscienze* (trans. R Lucchi, A Poli, M Virgili). Zanichelli, Bologna.

Rice DP (ed.). (2008) *Craniofacial sutures. Development, disease and treatment.* Karger, London.

Schindler O, Ruoppolo G, Schindler A (eds). (2011) *Deglutologia*, 2nd edn. Omega Edizioni, Turin.

Serrano MJ, So S, Hinton RJ. (2014) Roles of notch signaling in mandibular condylar cartilage. *Arch Oral Biol* 59(7), 735–740.

Simoes W (ed.). (2013) *Jaw functional orthopedics. TMD and orofacial pain.* TOTA Ribeirao Preto, Sao Paolo.

Slavicek R. (2002) *The masticatory organ: functions and dysfunctions.* Gamma Medizinisch-wissenschaftliche Fortbildung-AG, Klosterneuburg.

Stevens K, Bressmann T, Gong SG, Tompson BD. (2011) Impact of a rapid palatal expander on speech articulation. *Am J Orthod Dentofacial Orthop* 140(2), e67–e75.

Thilander B, Bjerklin K. (2012) Posterior crossbite and temporomandibular disorders (TMDs): need for orthodontic treatment? *Eur J Orthod* 34(6), 667–673.

Thilander B, Carlsson GE, Ingervall B. (1976) Postnatal development of the human temporomandibular joint. I. A histological study. *Acta Odontol Scand* 34(2), 117–126.

Throckmorton GS, Buschang PH, Hayasaki H, Pinto AS. (2001) Changes in the masticatory cycle following treatment of posterior unilateral crossbite in children. *Am J Orthod Dentofacial Orthop* 120(5), 521–529.

Chapter 6

Cases

Contents

Understanding Masticatory Function in Unilateral Crossbites, First Edition. Maria Grazia Piancino and Stephanos Kyrkanides.
© 2016 John Wiley & Sons, Inc. Published 2016 by John Wiley & Sons, Inc.

6.1 Introduction

This chapter is dedicated to the presentation of seven significant cases of crossbite.

The cases presented show the results obtained with the FGB, in everyday practice, for the correction of both crossbite malocclusion and masticatory function at different stages of development. The cases are documented with photographs of the face and occlusion, orthopantomography, X-ray teleradiographies and cephalometries, and possibly chewing cycles. The increase of the intermolar distance as measured by calipers and its stability or improvement after correction are shown by photographs of casts of the palate. It must be pointed out that the intermolar distance is a linear measurement and does not show the real improvement obtained by the FGB in the three planes of the space, especially the improvement of the asymmetry of the palate, for which a 3D cone-beam could be useful (although this is not recommended during therapy at an early age for radioprotection reasons).

All cases are presented before therapy, after correction, and at different follow-up stages. The improvement of the intermolar distance demonstrated at follow-up is not only stable but continues to improve. This is due to the fact that, as explained in Chapter 4, after correction, it is important to continue using the appliance during the night as an active physiological retention. The FGB appliance does not have a dental anchorage, and so the teeth and the supporting bones are free to grow; in this way it is able to adapt to the growing structures and to the permanent dentition, continuously self-repositioning the mandible and the growing condyles in the most centered position, maintaining the leveling of the occlusal plane and the alignment of the dental arches, transmitting self-regulated intermittent forces where needed and encouraging the bone growth with the decompression spaces. The FGB appliance works in respect of the biology and physiology of the structures of the stomatognathic system. It is a true gnathological appliance.

6.2 Case 1: Right unilateral posterior crossbite (3 years, 9 months)

This case examines a right unilateral posterior crossbite with functional shift in a boy aged 3 years and 9 months.

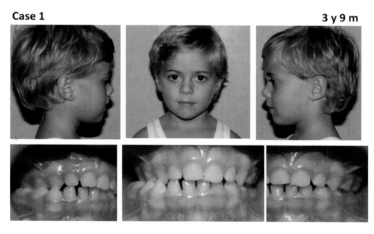

Figure 6.1 *Top:* images of the face; *bottom:* images of the occlusion (frontal and lateral views). The X-ray and cephalometric analyses were not performed owing to the very young age of the patient. They will be requested at a later stage in development.

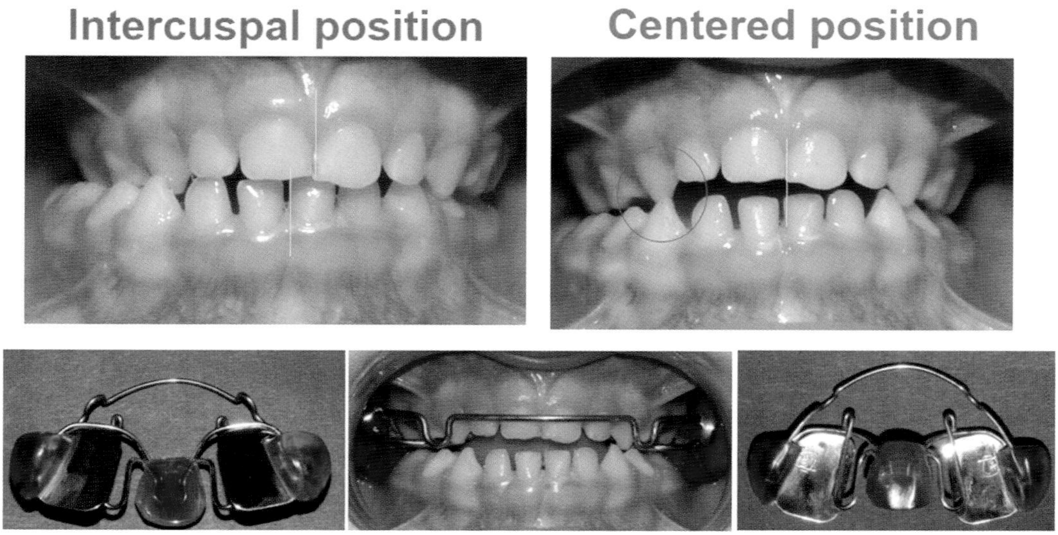

Intercuspal position   Centered position

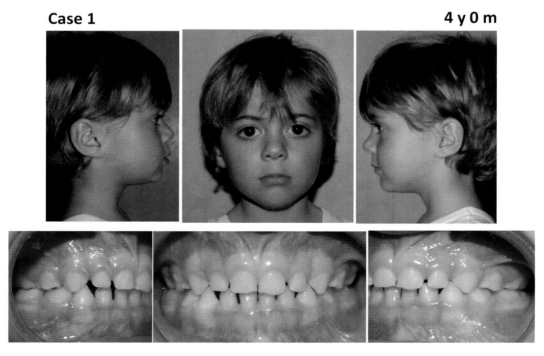

Figure 6.2 *Top:* maximum intercuspal position (on the left) and centered position with centered midlines (on the right). Observe the occlusal incongruence. *Bottom:* view of the FGB appliance in the mouth and out of the mouth (view of the lower side of the appliance on the left, and of the upper side on the right). As soon as the FGB appliance is in the mouth, the mandible is centered.

Case 1   **4 y 0 m**

Figure 6.3 Images of the face (*top*) and of the occlusion (*bottom*) after 3 months of therapy with FGB.

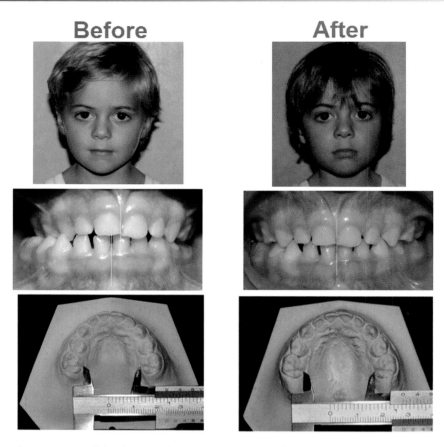

Figure 6.4 Comparison of the face, occlusion, and palate before (*left*) and after (*right*) correction of the unilateral posterior crossbite. The intermolar distance measured with a caliper on the stonecasts shown in the image was 2.5 cm before and 2.9 cm after correction (increase of 4 mm).

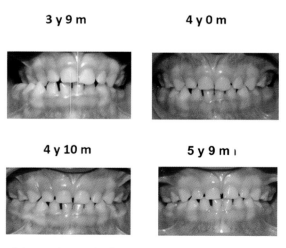

Figure 6.5 Comparison of the occlusion before therapy (3.9 y), after correction (4.0 y), at 10 months (4.10 y) and at 21 months (5.9 y) follow-up (FGB appliance was worn during the night).

6.3 Case 2: Right unilateral posterior crossbite (6 years, 4 months)

This case examines a right unilateral posterior crossbite in a girl aged 6 years and 4 months.

Case 2   **6 y 4 m**

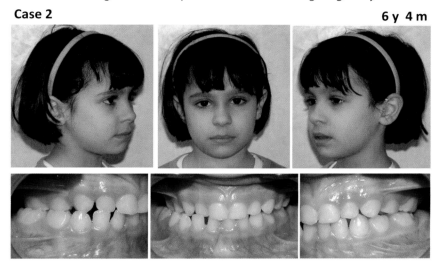

Figure 6.6   *Top:* images of the face; *bottom:* images of the occlusion (frontal and lateral views).

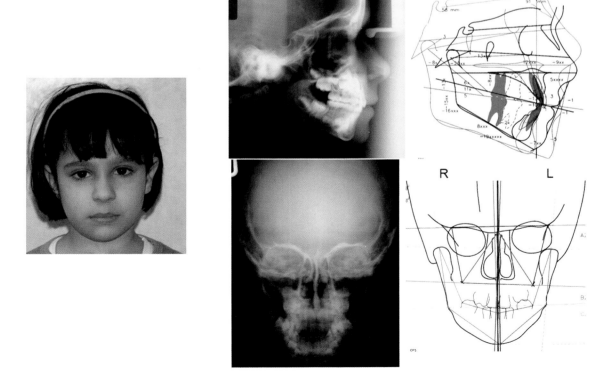

Figure 6.7   Latero-lateral and postero-anterior teleradiography (*left*) and cephalometric tracings (*right*).

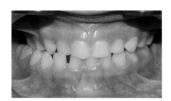

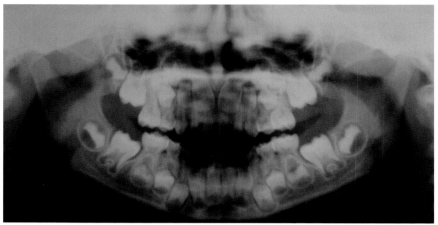

Figure 6.8 Maximal intercuspation (*top*) and orthopantomography (*bottom*).

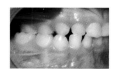

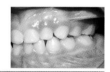

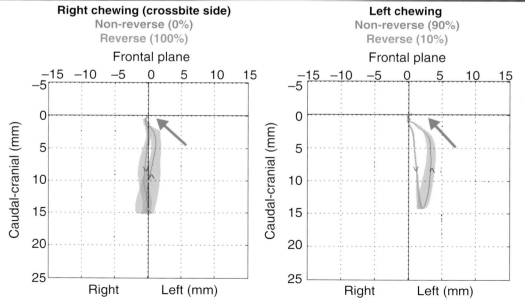

Figure 6.9 Chewing cycles before therapy; observe the severe alteration of the pattern morphology during chewing on the crossbite side and the consequent serious functional asymmetry.

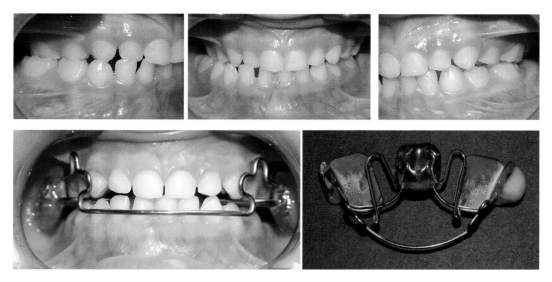

Figure 6.10 Maximal intercuspation (*top*) and FGB appliance in the mouth and out of the mouth (*bottom*). Observe the asymmetric activation of the buccal shields.

Case 2   6 y 8 m

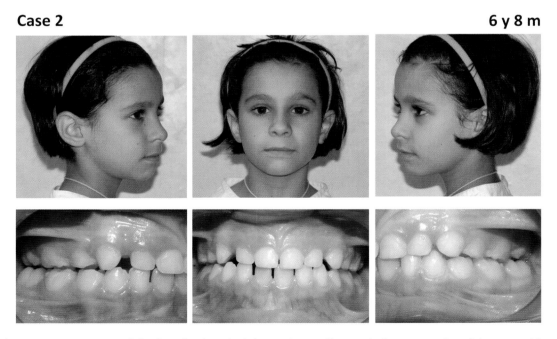

Figure 6.11 Images of the face (*top*) and of the occlusion (*bottom*) after 4 months of therapy with the FGB appliance.

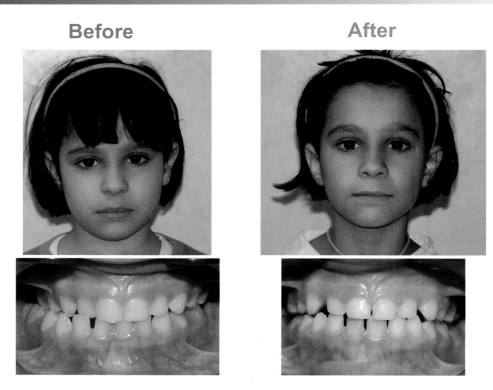

Before

After

Figure 6.12 Comparison of the face and occlusion before (on the left) and after correction of the unilateral posterior crossbite (on the right).

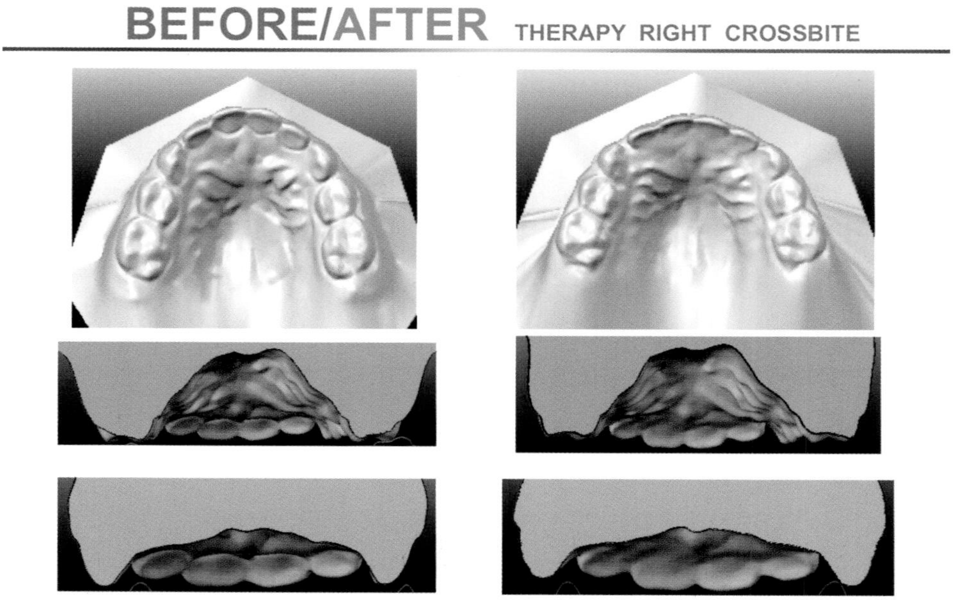

BEFORE/AFTER THERAPY RIGHT CROSSBITE

Figure 6.13 Comparison of the e-models of palate before and after correction of the right unilateral posterior crossbite.

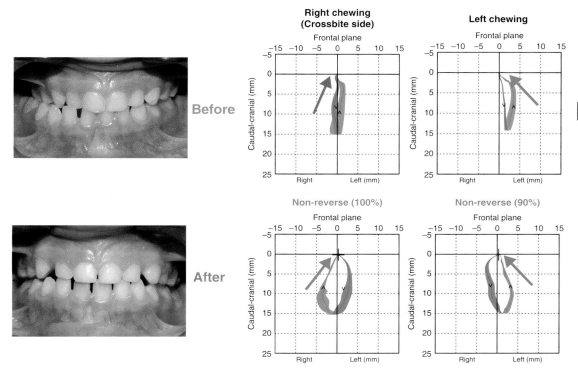

Figure 6.14 Comparison of the chewing cycles before (*top*) and after correction of the right unilateral posterior crossbite (*bottom*). Observe the recovery of the functional symmetry.

6.4 Case 3: Positional crossbite (7 years, 6 months)

This case examines a right unilateral posterior crossbite with functional shift in a boy aged 7 years and 6 months with primary dentition.

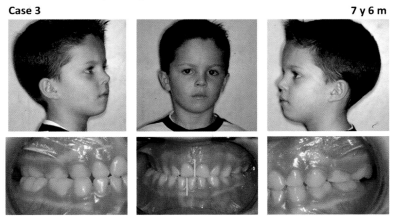

Figure 6.15 *Top:* images of the face; *bottom:* images of the occlusion (frontal and lateral views).

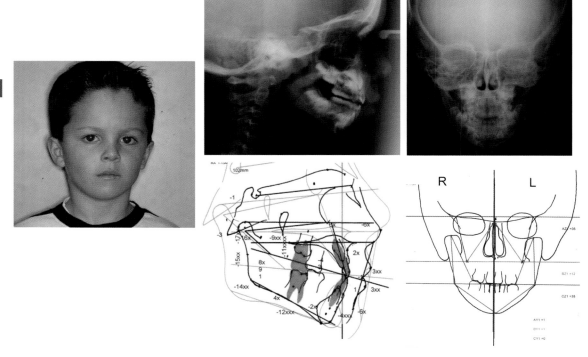

Figure 6.16 *Top:* latero-lateral and postero-anterior teleradiography recorded with the mandible in centered position. *Bottom:* cephalometric tracings. Observe the hyperdivergent tendency.

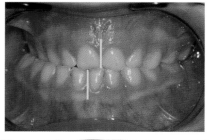

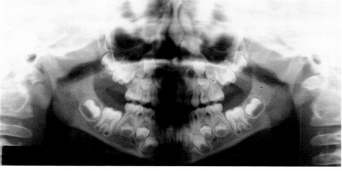

Figure 6.17 Maximal intercuspation (*top*) and orthopantomography (*bottom*).

Intercuspal position

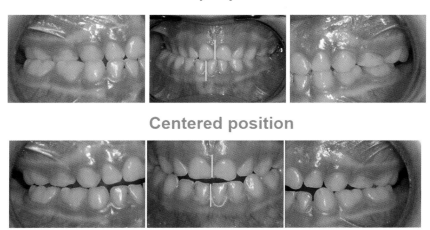

Centered position

Figure 6.18 Comparison of intercuspal position (*top*) and centered position (*bottom*). Observe the cusp-to-cusp contacts in centered position.

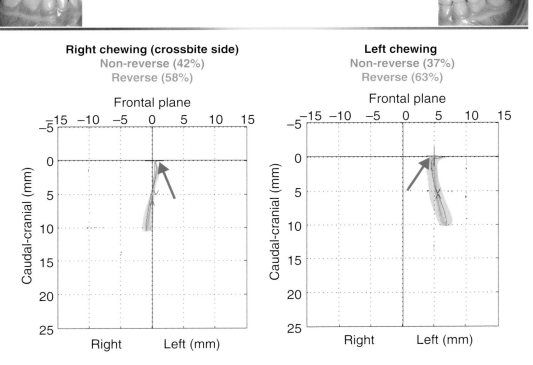

Right chewing (crossbite side)
Non-reverse (42%)
Reverse (58%)

Left chewing
Non-reverse (37%)
Reverse (63%)

Figure 6.19 Chewing cycles before therapy. Observe the severe alteration of the pattern morphology during chewing on both sides due to the occlusal instability represented by the different position of the functional intercuspation (see Section 2.3).

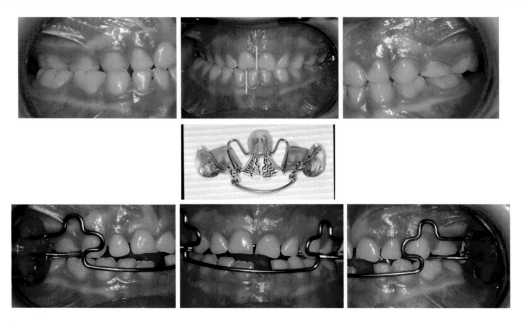

Figure 6.20 Images of the occlusion without (*top*) and with (*bottom*) the FGB appliance. When the appliance is in the mouth, the midlines are centered and the occlusion is protected from traumatic cusp-to-cusp contacts. The mandible is free to self-regulate the position in the three planes of space at any stage of therapy, thanks to the smooth stainless steel resilient bite planes. The self-regulated position of the mandible, free from dental contacts, enables the condyles to spontaneously find the most physiological position within the TMJ. In this way it is possible to avoid any type of joint compensation (see Section 2.3),as happens with traumatic and antiphysiological therapies.

Case 3   **7 y 10 m**

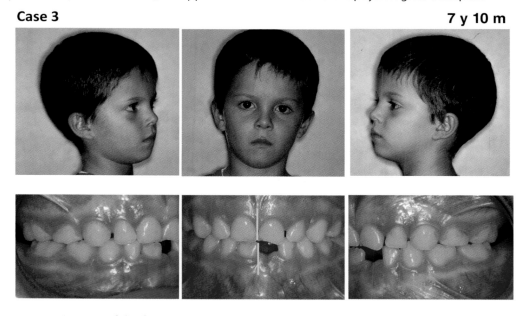

Figure 6.21 Images of the face (*top*) and of the occlusion (*bottom*) after 4 months of therapy with the FGB appliance.

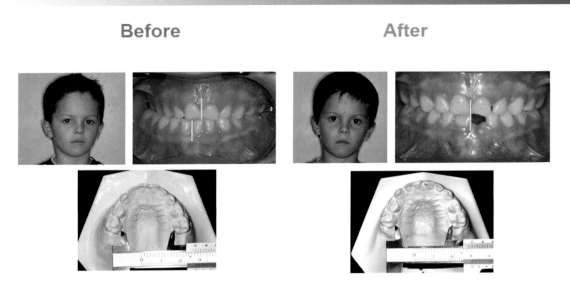

Figure 6.22 Comparison of the face, occlusion, and palate before and after correction of the unilateral posterior crossbite. The intermolar distance measured with a caliper on the stonecasts shown in the image was 2.9 cm before and 3.2 cm after correction (increase of 3 mm). Observe the arch form.

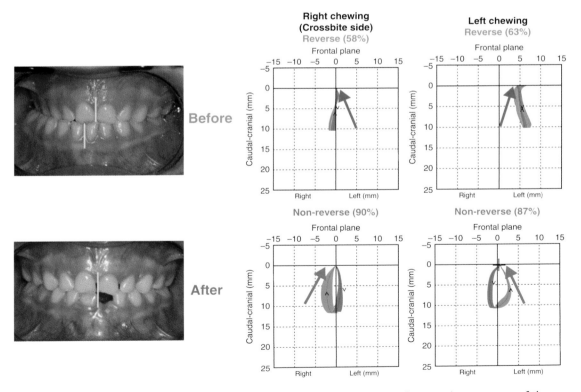

Figure 6.23 Chewing cycles before (*top*) and after therapy (*bottom*). Observe the recovery of the functional physiology and symmetry.

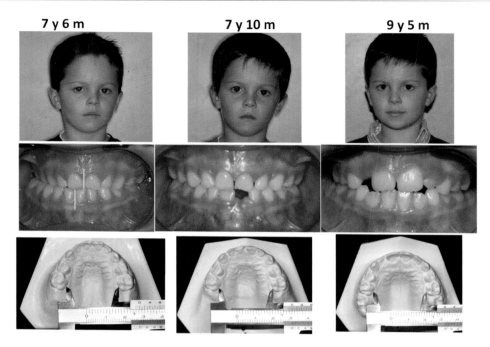

Figure 6.24 Comparison of the face, occlusion, and palate before therapy (*left*), after correction (*center*) and at 9.5 years of age (*right*). The intermolar distance measured with a caliper on the stonecasts shown in the image was 2.9 cm before, 3.2 cm after correction, and 3.35 cm at 2 years' follow-up (increase of 4.5 mm measured at the second deciduous molar). Observe the absence of relapse, the stability of the correction, and the continuous improvement of the intermolar distance and palatal shape.

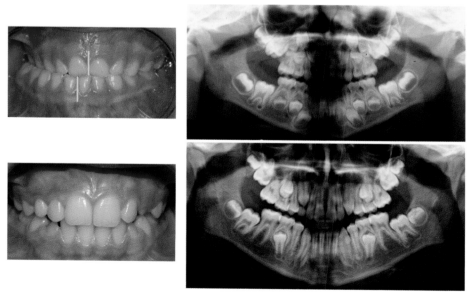

Figure 6.25 Maximal intercuspation and orthopantomography before (*top*) and after correction (*bottom*).

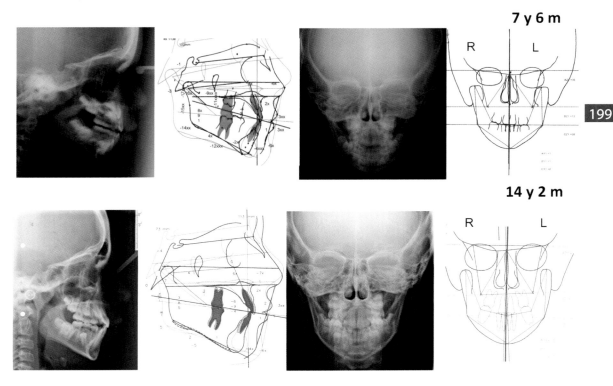

7 y 6 m

R   L

14 y 2 m

R   L

Figure 6.26 Latero-lateral and postero-anterior teleradiography and cephalometric tracings before (*top*) and after (*bottom*) correction of unilateral posterior crossbite, at age 14 years and 2 months.

FOLLOW UP   **14 y 2 m**

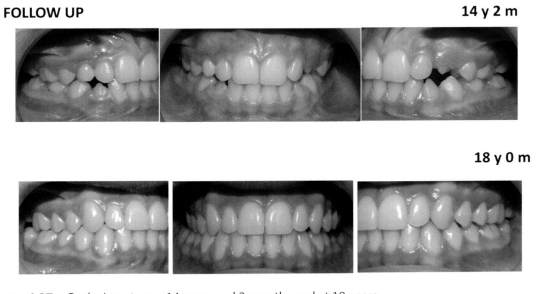

18 y 0 m

Figure 6.27 Occlusion at ages 14 years and 2 months and at 18 years.

6.5 Case 4: Left unilateral posterior crossbite (7 years, 11 months)

This case examines a left unilateral posterior crossbite in a boy aged 7 years and 11 months with mixed dentition.

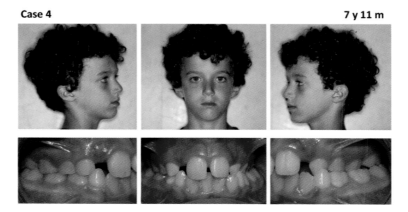

Figure 6.28 *Top:* images of the face; *bottom:* images of the occlusion (frontal and lateral views).

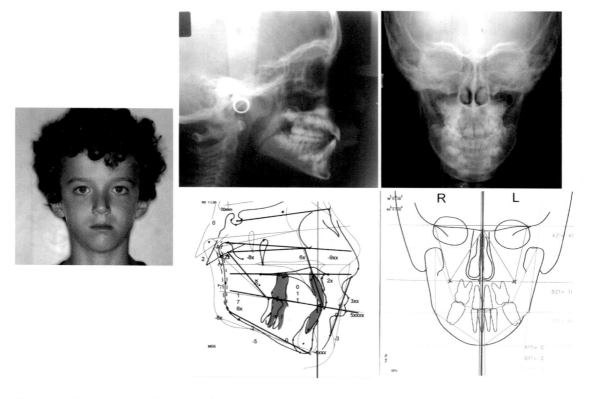

Figure 6.29 *Top:* latero-lateral and postero-anterior teleradiography. *Bottom:* cephalometric tracings.

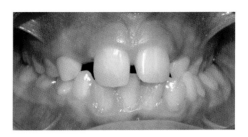

Figure 6.30 Maximal intercuspation and orthopantomography.

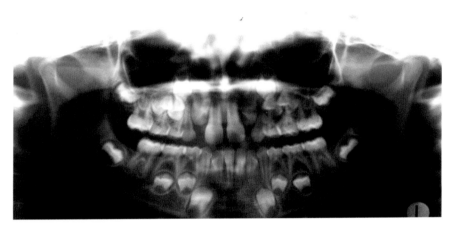

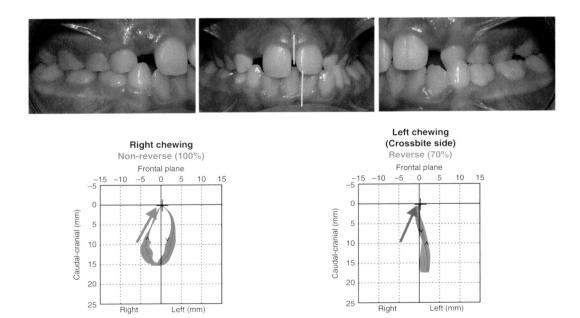

Figure 6.31 The chewing patterns before therapy. Observe the severe alteration of the pattern morphology during chewing on the crossbite side and the consequent serious functional asymmetry.

Case 4   **7 y 11 m**

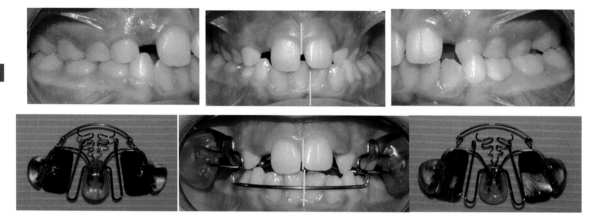

Figure 6.32   Images of the mouth without (*top*) and with the FGB appliance (*bottom*). When the appliance is in the mouth the mandible are centered. View of the lower side of the appliance (*right*) and of the upper side (*left*).

Case 4   **8 y 6 m**

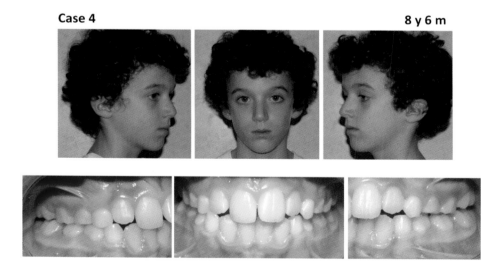

Figure 6.33   Images of the face (*top*) and of the occlusion (*bottom*) after 7 months of therapy with the FGB appliance.

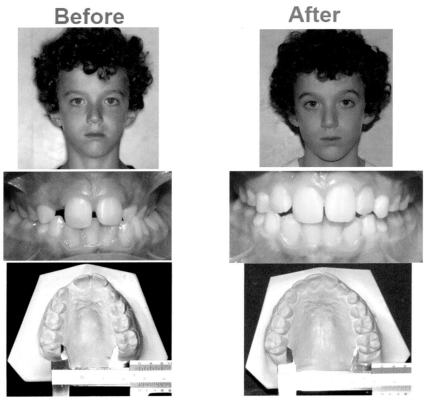

Figure 6.34 Comparison of the face, occlusion, and palate before therapy and after correction. The intermolar distance measured with a caliper on the stonecasts shown in the image was 2.9 cm before and 3.5 cm after correction (increase of 6 mm).

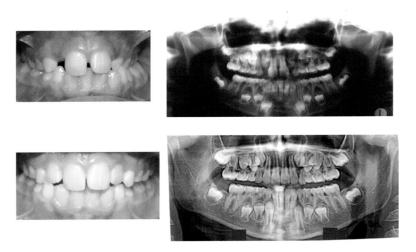

Figure 6.35 Maximal intercuspation and orthopantomography before (*top*) and after therapy with FGB (*bottom*).

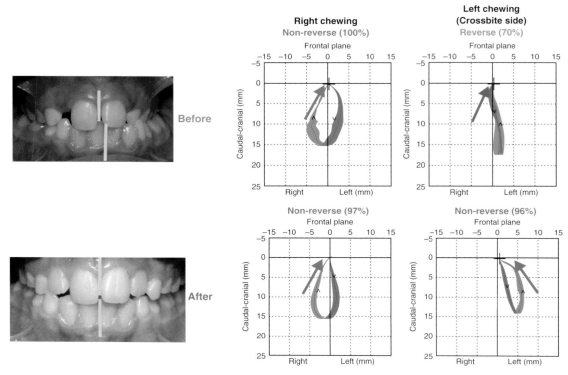

Figure 6.36 Chewing patterns before and after therapy. Observe the recovery of the functional physiology and symmetry of the chewing pattern.

Follow up   **10 y 6 m**

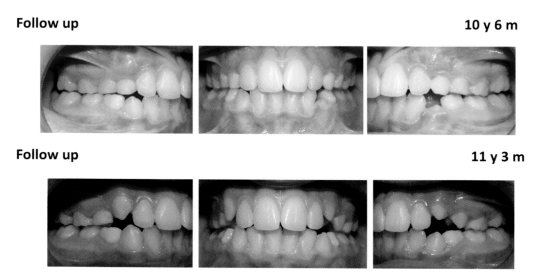

Follow up   **11 y 3 m**

Figure 6.37 Follow-up of the occlusion at ages 10 years and 6 months (*top*) and at 11 years and 3 months (*bottom*). The appliance FGB was worn as much as possible until the correction of crossbite and then at home and during the night.

6.6 Case 5: Right unilateral posterior crossbite (10 years, 3 months)

This case examines a right unilateral posterior dento-alveolar crossbite in a boy aged 10 years and 3 months with mixed dentition.

Case 5   **10 y 3 m**

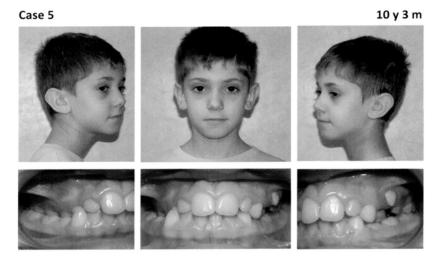

Figure 6.38 *Top:* images of the face; *bottom:* images of the occlusion (frontal and lateral views).

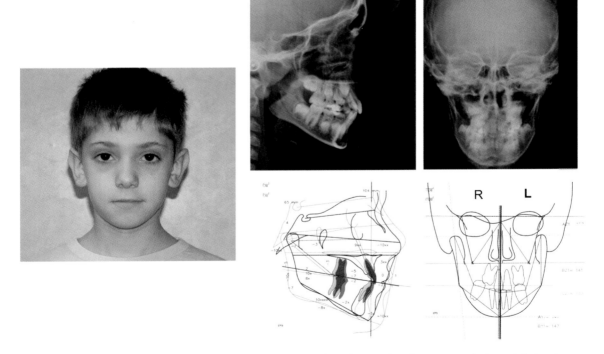

Figure 6.39 *Top:* latero-lateral and postero-anterior teleradiography. *Bottom:* cephalometric tracings.

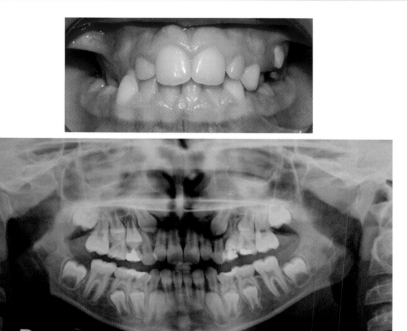

Figure 6.40 *Top:* maximal intercuspation; *bottom:* orthopantomography.

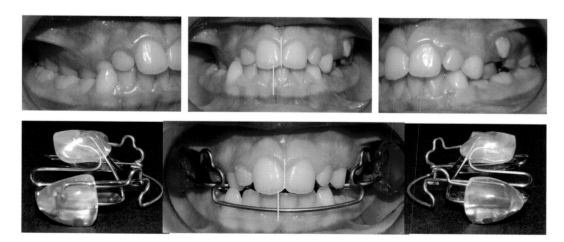

Figure 6.41 Images of the mouth without (*top*) and with (*bottom*) the FGB appliance.

Case 5

11 y 1 m

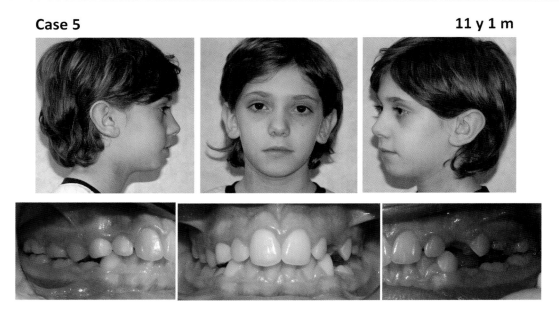

Figure 6.42   Images of the face (*top*) and of the occlusion (*bottom*) after 10 months of therapy with the FGB appliance.

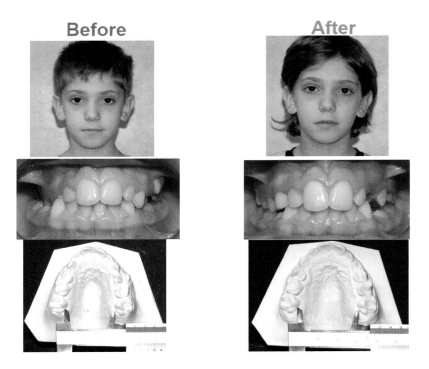

Figure 6.43   Comparison of the face, occlusion, and palate before and after correction of the unilateral posterior crossbite. The intermolar distance measured with a caliper on the stonecasts shown in the image was 2.9 cm before and 3.3 cm after correction (increase of 4 mm).

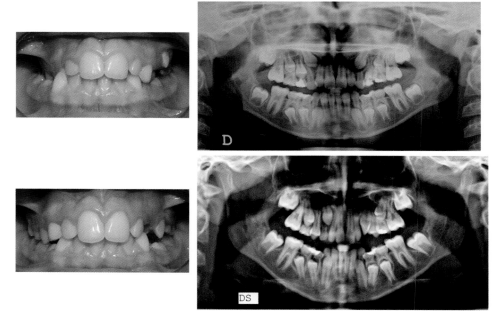

Figure 6.44 Comparison of the occlusion and orthopantomography before and after therapy.

FOLLOW UP   **13 y 0 m**

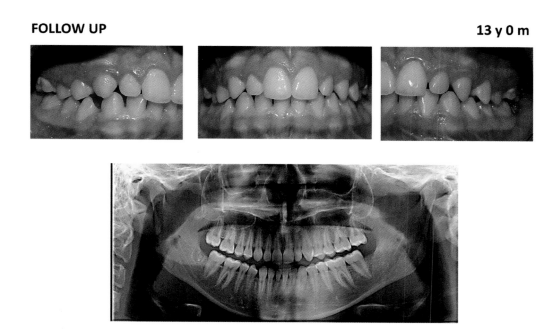

Figure 6.45 Images of the occlusion (*top*) and orthopantomography (*bottom*) at 2 years and 9 months' follow-up. Observe the parallelism of the roots due to the action of the resilient stainless steel bite planes.

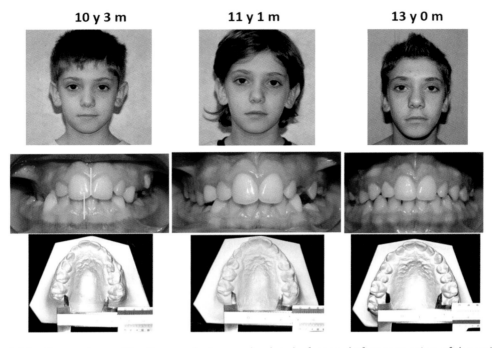

Figure 6.46 Comparison of the face, occlusion, and palate before and after correction of the unilateral posterior crossbite and at 13 years of age. Observe the improvement of the shape of the upper arch. The intermolar distance measured with a calipers on the stonecasts shown in the image was 2.9 cm before, 3.3 cm after correction, and 3.6 cm at 2 years and 9 months' follow-up (increase of 7 mm).

6.7 Case 6: Anterior open bite and left unilateral posterior crossbite (7 years, 9 months)

This case examines an anterior open bite and left unilateral posterior crossbite in a girl aged 7 years and 9 months with mixed dentition.

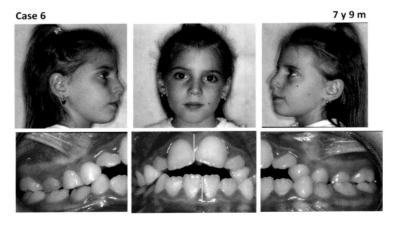

Figure 6.47 Images of the face (*top*); images of the occlusion (*bottom*) (frontal and lateral views).

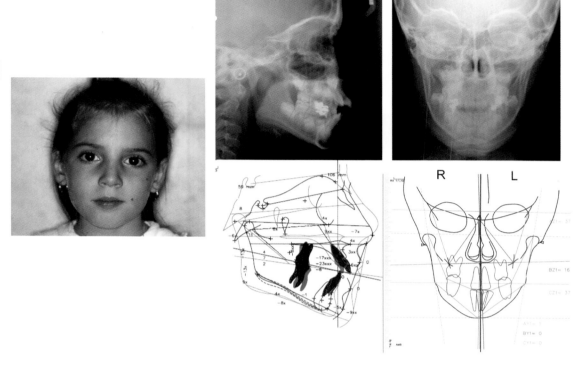

Figure 6.48 *Top:* latero-lateral and postero-anterior teleradiography. *Bottom:* cephalometric tracings.

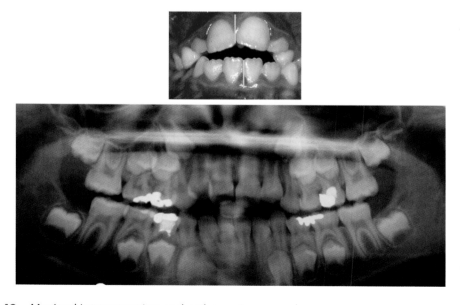

Figure 6.49 Maximal intercuspation and orthopantomography.

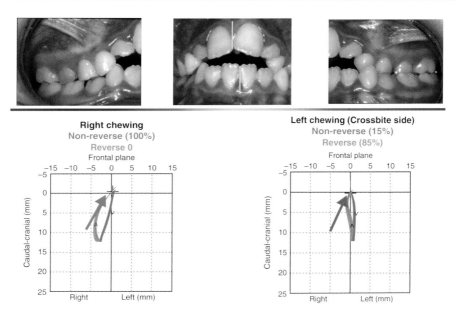

Figure 6.50 The chewing patterns before therapy of left posterior crossbite. Observe the severe alteration of the pattern morphology during chewing on the crossbite side (left side) and the consequent serious functional asymmetry.

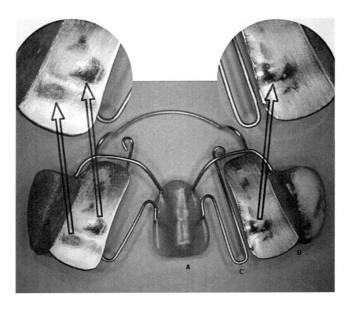

Figure 6.51 The FGB appliance.

Case 6   8 y 3 m

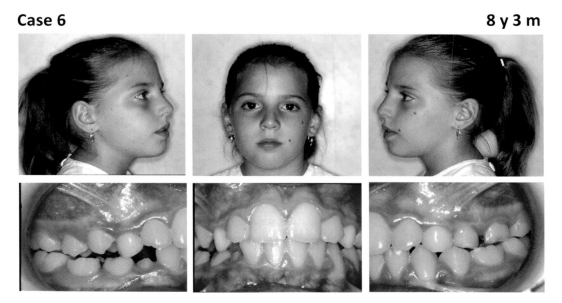

Figure 6.52 Images of the face (*top*) and of the occlusion (*bottom*) after 6 months of therapy with the FGB appliance.

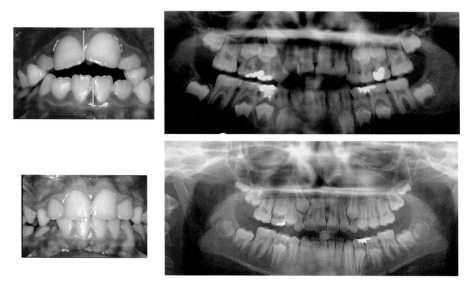

Figure 6.53 Occlusion and orthopantomography before and after correction of the anterior open bite and left posterior crossbite.

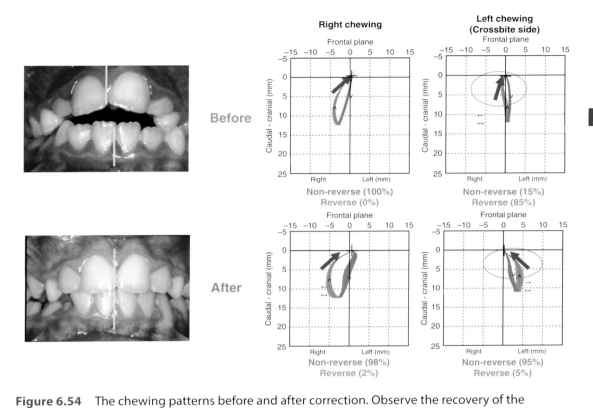

Figure 6.54 The chewing patterns before and after correction. Observe the recovery of the functional symmetry and of the closure direction.

Case 6   9 y 5 m

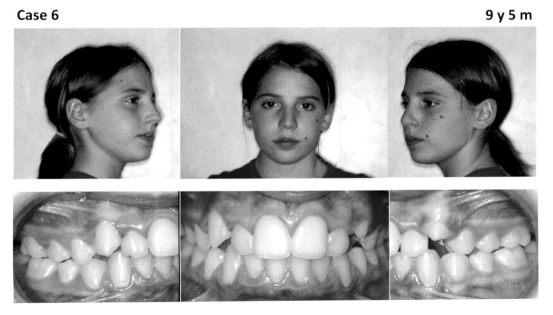

Figure 6.55 Image of face and occlusion at age 9 years and 5 months.

214

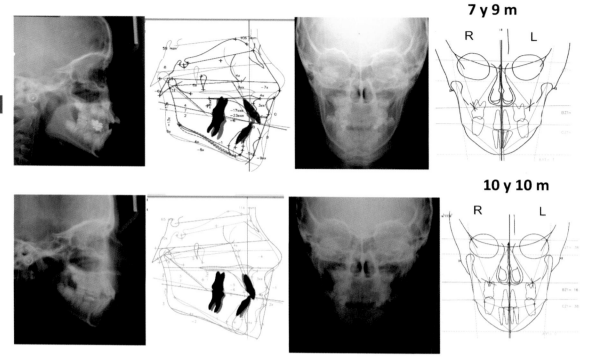

7 y 9 m

10 y 10 m

Figure 6.56 Latero-lateral and postero-anterior teleradiography and cephalometric tracings before (*top*) and at 10 years and 10 months (*bottom*).

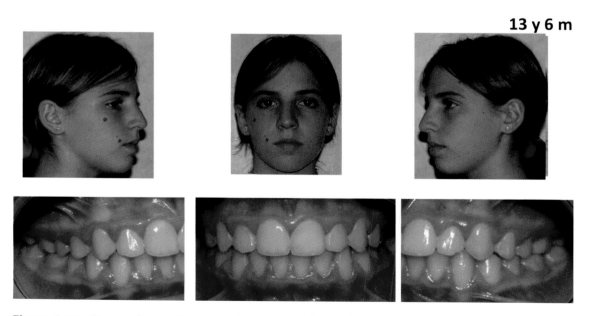

13 y 6 m

Figure 6.57 Face and occlusion at age 13 years and 6 months. In this case the aesthetic alignment has been obtained with a short period of fixed appliance (8 months).

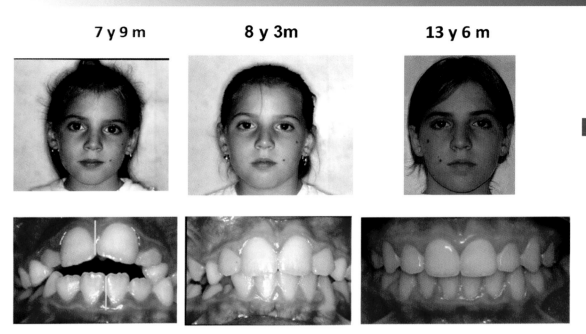

7 y 9 m   8 y 3m   13 y 6 m

Figure 6.58   Comparison of the face and occlusion before and after correction of the unilateral posterior crossbite and at age 13 years and 6 months.

6.8 Case 7: Anterior open bite and bilateral posterior crossbite (7 years, 8 months)

This case examines an anterior open bite and bilateral posterior crossbite in a girl aged 7 years and 8 months with mixed dentition. This is a severe malocclusion that has been presented to show the potentiality of the appliance and the progressive improvement of the masticatory function.

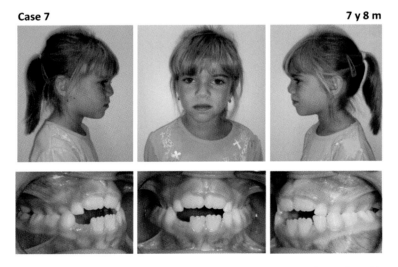

Case 7   7 y 8 m

Figure 6.59   *Top*: images of the face; *bottom:* images of the occlusion (frontal and lateral views).

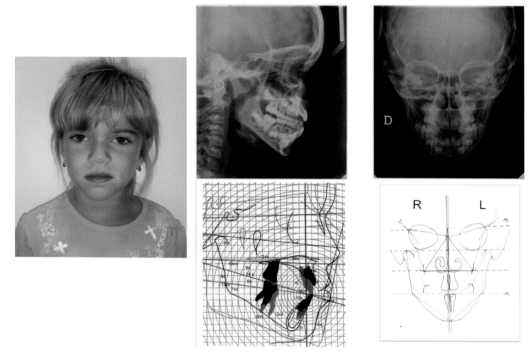

Figure 6.60 *Top:* latero-lateral and postero-anterior teleradiography. *Bottom:* cephalometric tracings. Observe the hyperdivergent tendency.

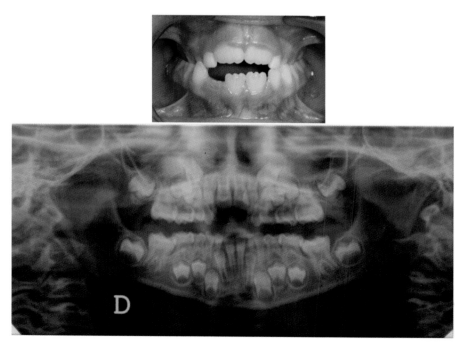

Figure 6.61 Maximal intercuspation and orthopantomography.

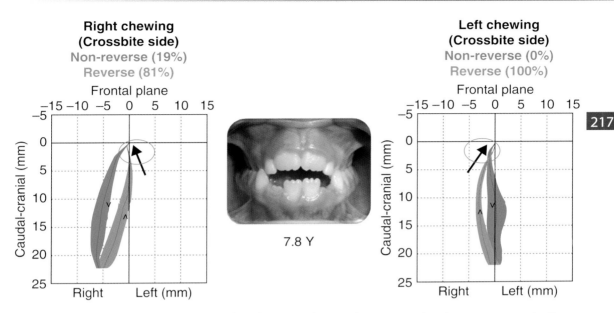

Figure 6.62 The chewing patterns before therapy. Observe the reverse chewing patterns on both sides.

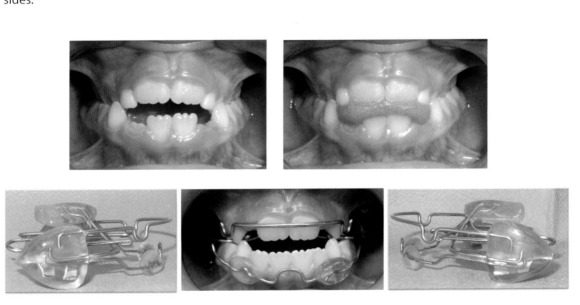

Figure 6.63 Images of the occlusion without (*top*) and with (*bottom*) the FGB appliance. Observe the alteration of the tongue function.

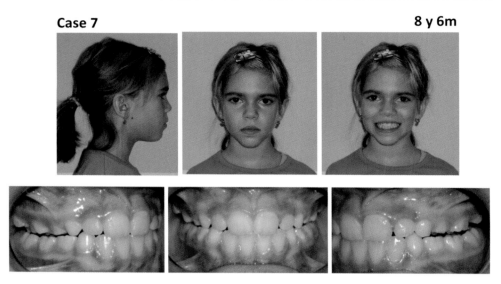

Case 7   **8 y 6m**

Figure 6.64   Images of the face (*top*) and of the occlusion (*bottom*) after 10 months of therapy with the FGB appliance.

Before   **After**

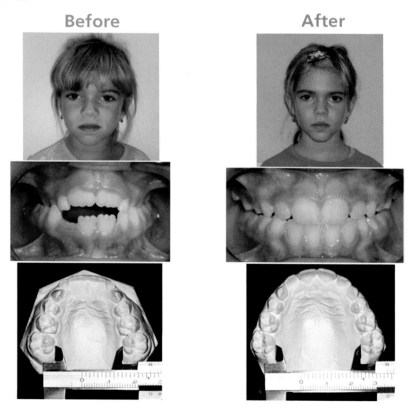

Figure 6.65   Comparison of the face, occlusion, and palate before and after correction of the bilateral posterior crossbite and anterior open bite. The intermolar distance measured with a caliper on the stonecasts shown in the image was 2.7 cm before and 3.6 cm after correction (increase of 9 mm).

FOLLOW-UP   **11 Y 3 M**

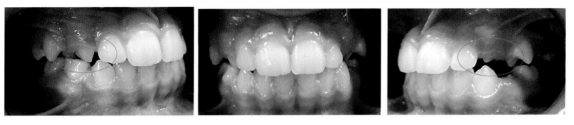

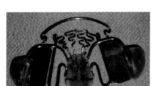

                                                                        12 Y 8 M

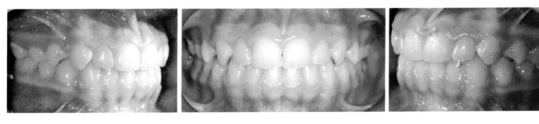

Figure 6.66 Image of occlusion at ages 11 years and 3 months (*top*), observe that both the upper right and left canine erupted in crossbite: they were easily and immediately corrected adapting the expansion spring, without any need of laboratory work and 12 years and 8 months (*bottom*). *Middle:* the FGB appliance.

7 y 8 m **8 y 6 m** **12 y 8 m**

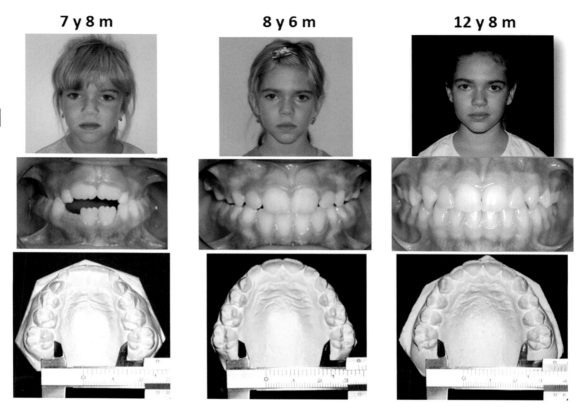

Figure 6.67 Comparison of the face, occlusion, and palate before (*left*) and after therapy (*center*) and at years and follow up (*right*). The intermolar distance measured with a caliper on the stonecasts shown in the image was 2.7 cm before correction, 3.6 cm after correction, and 3.7 cm at 5 years follow-up (increase of 10 mm). Observe the improvement of the arch form.

7 y 8 m   **10 y 0 m**   **12 y 8 m**

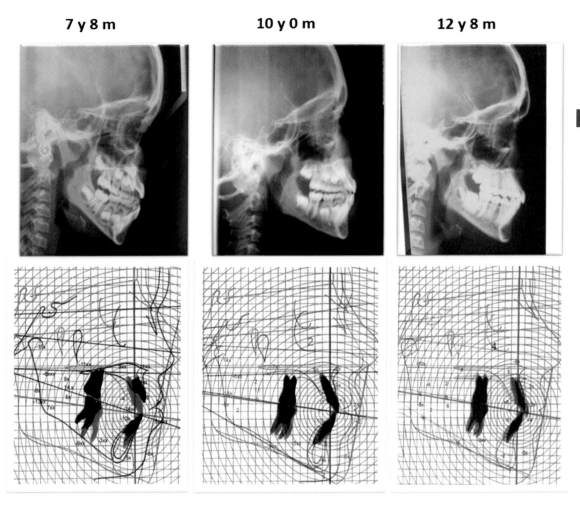

Figure 6.68   Latero-lateral teleradiography before therapy (*left*), at 10 years (*center*), and at 12 years and 8 months (*right*). *Bottom:* cephalometric tracings.

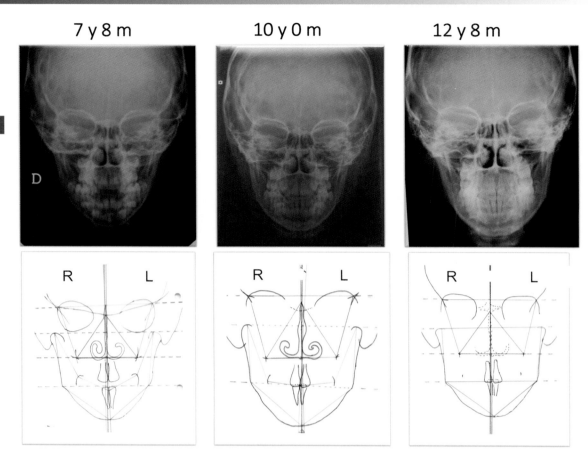

Figure 6.69 Postero-anterior teleradiography before therapy (*left*), at 10 years (*center*), and at 12 years and 8 months (*right*). *Bottom:* cephalometric tracings.

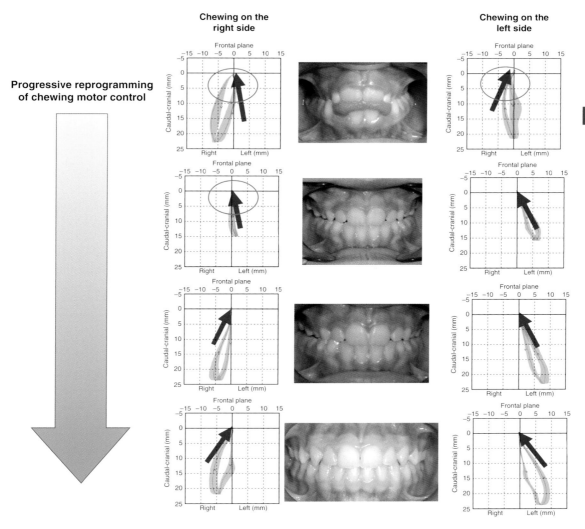

Figure 6.70 Progressive reprogramming of the chewing motor control, with the arrows representing the direction of the pattern of closure progressively restored. Observe the progressive improvement of the symmetry of the chewing pattern.

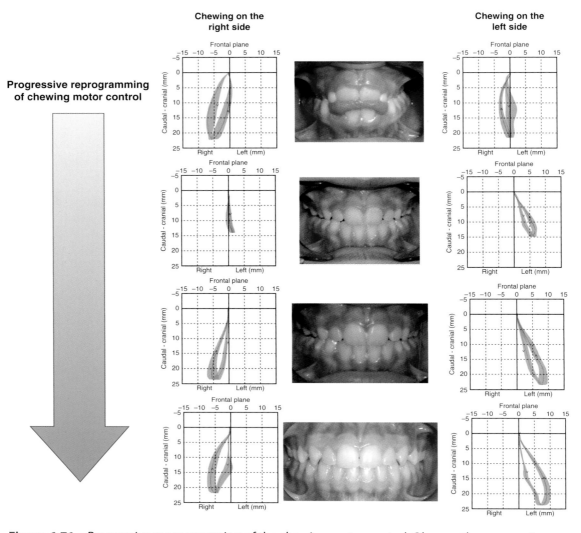

Figure 6.71 Progressive reprogramming of the chewing motor control. Observe the progressive improvement of the chewing pattern.

Appendix: Terminology Update

Use this page to add to/modify the terminology discussed in Chapter 2 (Section 2.3).

Index

Notes: Abbreviations used: FGB - function generating bite
Pages numbers in *italics* refer to figures

Understanding Masticatory Function in Unilateral Crossbites, First Edition. Maria Grazia Piancino and Stephanos Kyrkanides.
© 2016 John Wiley & Sons, Inc. Published 2016 by John Wiley & Sons, Inc.